D0919141

FLORIDA STATE
UNIVERSITY LIBRARIES

JUN 8 2000

TALLAHASSEE, FLORIDA

HEARING MANY VOICES

THE HAMPTON PRESS COMMUNICATION SERIES

Feminist Studies

Transforming Visions: Feminist Critiques in Communication Studies
Sheryl Perlmutter Bowen and Nancy Wyatt (eds.)

Black and White Women as Friends: Building Cross-Race Friendships
Mary W. McCullough

Hearing Many Voices
M.J. Hardman and Anita Taylor (eds.)

HEARING MANY VOICES

EDITED BY

M. J. HARDMAN
UNIVERSITY OF FLORIDA

ANITA TAYLOR
GEORGE MASON UNIVERSITY

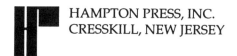
HAMPTON PRESS, INC.
CRESSKILL, NEW JERSEY

P
120
. W66
H 43
2000

Copyright © 2000 by Hampton Press, Inc.

All rights reserved. No part of this publication may be reproduced, stored in a retrieval system, or transmitted in any form or by any means, electronic, mechanical, photocopying, microfilming, recording, or otherwise, without permission of the publisher.

Printed in the United States of America

Library of Congress Cataloging-in-Publication Data

Hearing many voices / edited by M. J. Hardman, Anita Taylor.
    p. cm. -- (The Hampton Press communication series)
    Includes bibliographic references and index.
    ISBN 1-57273-237-7. -- ISBN 1-58273-238-5
    1. Women--Language. 2. Language and sex. I. Hardman,
Martha James. II. Taylor, Anita, 1935-. III. Series.
P120.W66H43 1999
408.2--dc21   99-42715
                                                                CIP

Hampton Press, Inc.
23 Broadway
Cresskill, NJ 07626

CONTENTS

v

PREFACE

We have stated in the introduction much that ordinarily would be included in a book preface. We edited this book (and planned the conference from which it grew) to give wider audience to a variety of women's voices that are too rarely heard. While in no case could we claim to have presented voices of all the women who should be heard, this book in its own small way does more of that than has other mainstream Western publishing. Our remaining hope is that what we have done will inspire or provoke more such publications and that we will encourage others to "listen" to the many voices that speak of women's experience, whether or not they are honored voices.

One matter relevant to the issues of hierarchical thinking that we discuss in the first chapter is the order in which editors' names are listed. Those of us who think in English incline to think the first listed name is the most important, the very principle that led us to write (and ask our authors to write) women and men, or she and he, whenever such constructions appear in our text. In our own work we try, not always successfully, to avoid implementing such a ranking principle. While each of us as editor (or author) has brought different strengths to this project, we have rarely worked in a situation in which a more balanced, equal, and egalitarian relationship existed. Truly, this book could not exist as it does without both of us. Thus, neither of us wishes to convey by the way our names appear that one of us has been more important to this book, or the introduction, than the other. Yet we know our English readers. For that reason, we are listed as editors with Hardman first, and as writers of the introduction with Taylor first.

Finally we want to state publicly our gratitude to those who have made this work possible. We thank especially our patient authors who endured delays and seemingly endless revisions and editing suggestions; Hampton Press publisher Barbara Bernstein; our series editor Brenda Dervin; and Dimas Bautista Iturrizaga, who did much to sustain body, mind, and soul as we struggled through the editing process.

CONTRIBUTORS

Sylvia L. Ashwell earned her master's degree in applied linguistics at the University of Florida in Gainesville. Her current research interests include cross-cultural communication, neurolinguistics, and autism, leading her to pursue a Ph.D. in psycholinguistics.

Leilani Cook completed her Ph.D. in 1995 and currently lives and works in Gainesville, Florida, where she writes about magical language and other sociolinguistic issues.

Mushira Eid is a professor in the Department of Languages and Literature and the Middle East Center at the University of Utah in Salt Lake City. Her research and teaching interests include Arabic linguistics, language and gender and code-switching.

LaTasha LaJourn Farmer was a student at the University of Florida when she prepared this paper.

Deborah Foreman-Takano, associate professor of English at Doshisha University, Kyoto, has been teaching English in Japan for 26 years. Her research concerns the cultural impact on various aspects of spoken language.

Patricia Geesey is associate professor of French and foreign cultures at the University of North Florida in Jacksonville. Her research interests include French-language fiction from North Africa, and Islam and North African immigration in France.

Dominique M. Gendrin is an Adjunct Faculty in Liberal Arts and Management Studies as the Culinary Institute of America in Poughkeepsie, NY. Her research focuses on cognition processes in various social groups.

Louise Gouëffic is executive director of Language Reform International (formerly, The Language Abuse Institute). She has recently published *Breaking the Patriarchal Code* (Manchester, CT: KIT, Knowledge, Ideas and Trends, Inc.).

Joan Kelly Hall is an associate professor in the Department of Language Education and a member of the Interdisciplinary Linguistics Program at the University of Georgia. Her research interests include the study of face-to-face second language learning contexts and intercultural communication.

M. J. Hardman is an professor of Linguistic Anthropology and a member of the Women's Studies Faculty at the University of Florida. She has specialized in the Aymara languages and in gender as it manifests itself in languages and cultures.

Mary R. Harmon is an associate professor of English at Saginaw Valley State University where she chairs the English Department. Her research interests include sociolinguistics and classroom discourse.

Yasuko Hio is a professor of English at the Shikoku Gakuin University in Zentsuji, Kagawa, Japan, where she has conducted research into gender patterns in Japanese.

Chieko Koyama is a Japanese student who completed a master's degree in anthropology at the University of Florida. She has been in the United States since 1994, and is interested in transformation of ethnic identity among Japanese-Brazilians who work as guest-workers in Japan.

David Natharius is a professor of communication and humanities at California State University, Fresno. His current research in gender issues includes examining role portrayals and archetypal images in film and literature.

Naoko Ogawa is an assistant professor of English at Kyoto Bunkyo College in Uji, Kyoto, Japan. She is also a Ph.D. candidate in linguistic anthropology at the University of California-Davis, currently working on her dissertation about gender indexing and gay male speech in Japan.

Lisa R. Perry was a student at the University of Florida when she prepared this paper.

Susan K. Shear is a graduate student in the Linguistic Program at the University of Florida. She specializes in the study of the Kannada language, Karnatak culture, and Lingayatism/Veerashaivism. She promotes understanding of this language, culture and philosophy through the development of websites sponsored by the Kogalur-Shear Corporation.

Anita Taylor is a professor of communication and member of the women's studies faculty at George Mason University, Fairfax, VA. Her research and teaching focus on communication ethics, persuasion, and gender in communication.

Lenora A. Timm is a professor of linguistics at the University of California, Davis, and director of the major program in nature and culture. Her research and teaching interests include bilingualism, minority languages, and language and gender.

Paola Traverso is currently working in Italy as a teacher trainer, specializing in young learners. She graduated in psychology at the Italian University of Padua and earned a Master's in speech communication from the University of Illinois at Urbana-Champaign.

INTRODUCTION:
THE MEANING OF VOICE

ANITA TAYLOR
M. J. HARDMAN

I am a feme[1]   not a fe+male
   I am a fem   not a wo+man
      I am a sapien   not a hu+man
I can name my self, therefore, I am a namer, and therefore, I must be a
critical thinker in the making of names, as well as in any other field of
thought. It is my right as a namer to name myself; no one else can
pretend to do so for me. To name me is to take my right of being a
thinker away from me.

   —Louise Gouëffic (this volume)

As man under fear of eternal damnation surrendered to the
irresponsible power of church and state, so woman yielded to that
power which closed every external avenue of knowledge to her under
pretext of her sinfulness.

---

[1]The terms *feme* and *fem* are historical words and were borrowed into Middle
English from French.

But woman is learning for herself that not self-sacrifice, but self-development, is her first duty in life; and this, not primarily for the sake of others but that she may become fully herself . . .
—Matilde Joslyn Gage, suffragist
Woman, Church & State (1893; cited in Wagner, 1980, p. 239)

Voices of women. How are they heard? Consider suffragist Matilde Joslyn Gage. Described in 1888 as one whose name, linked with Elizabeth Cady Stanton and Susan B. Anthony "will ever hold a grateful place in the hearts of posterity" (cited in Wagner, 1980, p. xv), by 1980 she merited eight "passing mentions," in four standard suffrage dictionaries, four with incorrect information (p. xxxviii). In contrast, Wagner found Anthony mentioned 168 times and Stanton 148 times.

For a long time, the story of the 19th-century women's rights movement was not taught in history books. By the late 1990s, that omission had been largely corrected, but the names that most people learn are those of Stanton and Anthony. Gage is known by few. Her voice has been almost entirely silenced.

Matilda Joslyn Gage was left by the wayside of history at least in part because she argued against the prevailing ideological system. She talked *with* the Iroquois, and could see that Native American women had what she did not. She described the position of Iroquois women as far superior to that of women in non-Indian nations:

> The famous Iroquois Indians, or Six Nations . . . showed alike in form of government, and in social life . . . women's superiority in power. . . . No sale of lands was valid without the consent of the squaws . . . and the Council of Matrons, to which all disputed questions were referred for final adjudication. . . . The women also possessed the veto power on questions of war. (Gage, 1893, p. 10)

Gage received the name of Ka-ron-ien-ha-wi or "She who holds the sky" when she was made an honorary member of the Iroquois wolf clan in 1893. She spoke out against the "oppression of Indians" and the breaking of treaties. She also concluded that the modern world was indebted to the Iroquois "for its first conception of inherent rights, natural equality of condition, and the establishment of a civilized government upon this basis" (Gage, 1893/1980, p. 10) because the constitution of the United States reflected that of the Six Nations Confederacy. Gage could envision a nation with such rights for all women, propounding these "radical" ideas at a time when movement leaders had turned in a more conservative direction, worrying about the "contamination" of their quest for the vote both by immigrants and Blacks. She became *persona non grata* among the women of the movement with her voice nearly completely lost to succeeding generations.

Consider as well Zora Neal Hurston. An anthropologist in the early part of the 20th century, she accomplished extraordinary feats considering how few women, and especially Black women, achieved any level of academic recognition during those years. Widely praised for her work by some of her contemporaries, Hurston persisted in working with language communities of poor and Black people. And she persisted in writing novels as well as "scholarship." The not surprising result is that she was unknown to succeeding generations as well until very recently (Washington, 1990).

What happened to those voices? How is it that we come to the end of the 20th century, after 30 years or more of feminist scholarship and activism and many well-educated people have heard of neither of these women, nor know anything of their work if they know the names? Why were Gage and Hurston, and many like them not heard, or if heard, not remembered?

The metaphor of voice and its recovery has been powerful in the 20th-century women's movement. Coming to realize we had voices that count and struggling to exercise those voices is in many ways "THE" story of this modern women's movement. We intend this book to serve as part of that struggle because it is motivated by the effort to hear a variety of women's voices. Our goal is to hear, record, and help others hear some of the breadth and strength of the voices of women often not heard.

In this introduction, we discuss the origins of the book, placing the work within the development of recent feminist scholarship in language, linguistics, and communication. We summarize the chapters included, attempting to show their relation to each other and to current scholarship. Finally, because we argue that it is important to understand the perspectives from which our own voices derive in order to be able to hear the voices of others, we end the introduction suggesting a variety of ways to "hear" these chapters despite the framing provided by our own thought systems.

Prior to Second Wave Feminism, the absence of women's voices pervaded our academic worlds. In the study of communication and speech, if one were to read the collections of "great" speeches, prior to 1960, one would think that no women gave speeches. And, listening to radio or watching television, it was well into the 1960s before women were heard in positive and active roles other than as entertainers. In linguistics, the study of language proceeded largely through study of the speech of men. When women's "register" was remarked on, it was to denigrate it by noting how weakly women talk and how trivial were the subjects to which they devoted attention. There was much study of the weighty talk of men, and only derision of the frivolous gossip of women, when they were not ignored entirely.

Our own areas of study were not alone in the dismissal of women, however. The 20th century has been described as the century in which the dominant religion changed from the church to that of psychology (Bellah, Madsen, Sullivan, Sidler, & Tipton, 1985). And in that change, we turned from a religion dominated by a male supernatural god to a discipline whose secular god (Freud) was at least as unkind to women. It was a long and difficult struggle, not finished yet, to rescue women from Freud and his disciples. Other areas of scholarship were little more welcoming to women. Before the 1960s, anthropology was almost exclusively the study of man and "his" cultures; sociology was the study of men in groups and social structures. Economics, which builds theories on which governments built policies, operated on the premise of the rational "man" who competes for scarce resources. As Tickner (1992) said, "Rational economic man is assumed to be motivated by the laws of profit maximization. He is highly individualistic, pursuing his own economic goals in the market without any social obligation to the community of which he is a part" (p. 72). History consisted largely of tales about governments, their armies, battles, treaties, laws, and efforts to control a populace. Few of those doing the governing were women; few women fought (or wanted to fight) in the armies; few negotiated the treaties or made the laws. There were some women in prominent places in business or government, but they were few and often achieved their position by inheriting a role or a business from a father or a politician husband who died in office. Even more rarely were their deeds chronicled to become part of history. In these circumstances, women understandably felt silenced.

Women were rarely in any roles of prominence anywhere in the public world. Many women worked outside the home, contrary to a widespread myth of today. But they worked in roles in which they were largely overlooked and in positions of relatively low influence. Women were domestics, cleaning staff, clerical workers, retail salespersons, garment workers, migrant laborers, nurses, nurses aides, elementary school teachers, and the like. They held positions that commanded low wages and equal amounts of respect.

DEVELOPMENT OF MODERN FEMINIST STUDY
ABOUT WOMEN AND LANGUAGE

Against this backdrop, the late 20th-century feminist movement of the United States rose out of the 20th-century civil rights movement and set itself to the task of putting women into roles of influence. Hearing the eloquent voices of the African-American struggle for freedom, we set out to reclaim our own voices—and to have them heard.

It was not long, however, before an incredible irony surfaced. We discovered our feminist movement itself guilty of silencing women's voices. Even women who spoke of alternate ways in which women's lives were being lived elsewhere were silenced, as though only the experience of one class of one race of women were relevant. This was the experience of one of the editors of this book, a feminist from the time she knew the word, but with no place in the movement until recently, because her work questioned early feminist orthodoxy.[2]

Perhaps the first to call themselves to our attention were African Americans. Using the words of Sojourner Truth, *Ain't I a Woman*, hooks (1981) wrote of being silenced in her classrooms at Stanford, but she was far from the only Black person who experienced the phenomenon or wrote about it (Davis, 1981; Hull, Scott, & Smith, 1982). And more than African Americans were involved. Only 3 years after being created, the National Organization for Women (NOW) nearly foundered over visibility of support for lesbians. Lesbians were welcome, indeed in many places were the backbone of women's groups, but they were urged to remain silent and invisible "for the good of the whole." During the first years of the movement, concerns of the poor seldom received high priority from women's groups. In both theory and practice, the 1960s and early 1970s women's "liberation" movement worked for goals the achievement of which would have little direct effect in improving the lot of the poor. Other minorities, whose interests often coincided with those of the poor, also found little benefit from the mainstream women's movement. Accurately accused of being primarily a White, middle-class movement, many of its members not only did not hear voices different from their own, but did not particularly *want* to hear

---

[2]As an example, much of the ethnographic data in Hardman (1994) was gathered some 20 or 30 years before the publication, and then only in 1994 did The Organization for the Study of Communication Language and Gender make publication of it possible. Contributions have been rejected even from feminist publications/conferences because the information I provided about the Jaqi women did not fit the canon. One article (Hardman, 1978) was delayed by several years in its publication for the same reason. Many others have yet to come into the public eye.

those voices. The accusations never accurately described all early 20th-century feminists; the description of the results was largely accurate. Voices of African-American women or Latinas or Native Americans, or those descended from Asian or Pacific Islanders were rarely heard. When the concerns of poor women were addressed, it was usually by someone speaking for them; we rarely heard them speak for themselves; we rarely made such forums available. The international voices heard were Anglo and European. Intellectual feminism was heard, but it was English and European.

Moreover, our work suffered from a distressing tendency to essentialize the idea of woman. All too often, we assumed that all (or at least most) women had common interests, common attitudes, common traits and dispositions. We talked and wrote as if what we knew about relatively small groups of white women was, therefore, true of other women. We behaved as if what we had in the English-speaking world, especially Canada, England, and the United States, was what everyone else would obviously look up to and want. When we were not ignoring them altogether, we were often patronizing when talking about or interacting with non-Western women.

Fortunately, our feminism was sufficiently deep that we did at last listen when others said, "Wait, you do not speak for me!" Beginning with the 1980s and increasingly in the late 1990s, feminism matured and developed until, in 1998, it included a wide variety of voices and resisted the overgeneralizing of the 1960s. We have a long way to go. Just as in the late 1990s, too few women's voices of any kind were heard in the public sphere, so too were too few not White, not privileged women's voices heard within the feminist movement. Not in our theory, our organizations, or our scholarship do we sufficiently represent the vast diversity of women's experiences and interests. But at least we realize that we do not. And it was just such a realization that led, first to a conference, and then to this book.

M. J. Hardman conceived the idea for the conference, "Our Own and Others' Voices" as a forum for many voices, out of her frustrating experiences finding a place in which persons other than White men could be heard. As conference director, she sought widely for a variety of participants, dispersed geographically as well as by cultural group and interests.[3] Growing from the conference, at which were heard many voices unfamiliar to the ears of English speakers with often surprising messages, was the idea that these should have a wider audience. These

---

[3]The two voices mentioned, of Matilde Joslyn Gage and Zora Neale Hurston were heard at the conference through the medium of monodrama performances by Sally Roesch Wagner and Phyllis McEwen Taylor, thereby breaking their silence, at least in part, and giving us voices across time as well as geography.

voices often question our assumptions about the nature of human "nature," and they require us to think again about our assumptions about diversity.

We invited many of those who presented at the conference to submit their papers for this volume and have interacted with the authors in an extensive editing process. Reconstructing our assumptions about the nature of human "nature," and rethinking our assumptions about diversity is a difficult process. Those of us who believed in the 1960s that we could build a nonracist and nonsexist society by deciding to do so never imagined how much time it would take. Therefore, even though it seems a long time since these chapters were first written, little in the book is susceptible to becoming dated. Most of what is here is timeless in that it gives the reader an idea of the variety of women's voices that can be heard. No one volume could ever include all possible voices. However, we have achieved some degree of diversity in the voices to include. Geographically, the contributions speak to some aspect of women and language in Japan, southern India, Santa Domingo, Italy, France, and Egypt, as well as Canada and the United States. In terms of language, we hear the voices of Cherokee, Kannada, Japanese, Spanish, Arabic, Black English, Italian, and French among others.

Having gathered a rich variety of contributions, we then faced the task of framing. We have chosen a format that, as far as we are able, provides a forum for the voices such that we the editors do not speak for the authors, and that the chosen authors do not speak for women not chosen from within their own cultures. All of us have tried to remain alert to avoid speaking for women in cultures not represented. We hope, through our framing, to help readers make sense of the whole. We have tried to do this, as mentioned, by utilizing the metaphor of voice. Later, we discuss groupings by the geography of the subjects, whether persons or language; and we also suggest alternative perspectives for viewing the whole.

THE VOICES IN THIS BOOK

Anytime one combines seventeen chapters representing almost as many diverse cultural viewpoints, any category system used to relate the pieces to each other and the whole includes elements that are artificial. Categories are created by the categorizer. So we here need to share why we arrange these chapters as we do.

We have built this book around the hearing of women's voices. Among the most productive uses of this metaphor of voice was when

Kramarae (1981) and Spender (1980) applied the muted group theory to women (E. Ardener, 1975; S. Ardener, 1975). Muted group theory, as developed by the Ardeners, describes what happens when dominant groups coexist in a society or culture with dominated groups. The dominant group, having the power, makes all the rules and enforces them, thus "muting" the subordinate group voices. The subordinate group has little influence (voice) in deciding what the rules will be or to whom they will be applied, and so on. The group and its voice are muted.

Kramarae (1974, 1981) and Spender (1980) pointed out that in patriarchal cultures, men are the dominant group, women the dominated. Men, having positions of public power, make the cultural rules and establish the means of enforcement. Kramarae and Spender extended the argument to communication. They claimed that, by and large, men created languages. This, Spender argued, is especially true of English because it was formalized by clerics and academics (and often these were the same person as clerics were the professors) who established rules for using English. Since women were not involved in formalizing the language, and were dominated in the culture that created it, Kramarae hypothesized, it does not serve them well. English does not name concepts important to women but to men (e.g., one can have a "seminal" idea; but was one ever described as "ovular"?). English also devalues concepts important to women but not to men (again, the "seminal" idea is an example; if one nurtured or incubated an idea it would have quite a different feeling, as would ovulating it). English uses male referents and terms (e.g., the "generic" he and the conclusion that number is more important than gender for the third-person indefinite pronoun). And there are, of course, many other examples that can be given to illustrate how the English language serves men and men's interests better than women (see Hill, 1986; Miller & Swift, 1976; Penelope, 1990). Thus, Kramarae concluded, to describe English as "muting" women is appropriate.

Elgin, following up on Kramarae's muted group theory, as a thought experiment constructed the fictional language Láadan to express women's perceptions more adequately than existing human languages as far as she and the theorists then knew. She wrote a science fiction novel, *Native Tongue* (1984), in which a group of linguist women constructed Láadan, and began using it so that it could become the native tongue for the children. One of the characters was especially talented in the construction of "lexicalizations"—the invention of terms for expressing concepts. An example of these terms is *radama* "to nontouch; to actively refrain from touching" and a word derived from that one, *radamalh* which means the same, but with evil intent (with the suffix ("lh"). Laadan has 11 roots that translate to "love" in English, for example, *ab* means "love for one liked but not respected"; *ad* is "love for one respected but not liked"; *éeme* "love for one neither liked nor respected"; *ashon* is "love for one not related by blood, but kin of the heart"; *azh* means "love for one sexually desired now"; and so on through as many varieties as eventual native speakers of Láadan may feel needed. *Native Tongue* and its sequels *Judas Rose* (1987) and *Earthsong* (1994) deal with the effects of such language use on perception and living. Other cultures could also be considered (e.g., Brantenberg, 1985). Some of these are represented in this book in terms of how language and women's status interact.

Russ (1983), also a science fiction author whose work is gender bending, shows *How to Suppress a Woman's Writing*, a set of discourse patterns that effectively deny women agency. In the last part of this chapter, we use Russ's set of discourse strategies for muting women's voices to discuss the chapters in this book.

Muted group theory is introduced here because the chapters in this volume are framed in terms of muting. The metaphor works because voices are muted in a variety of ways. *Mute* can mean to silence completely, as with the remote control for a television set or in the case of an autistic child. *Mute* can mean to soften the voice, as does the pedal on a piano. And *mute* can mean to change (distort) the sound, as does the hat used by a jazz trombonist or trumpeter. We see those kinds of muting in the groups to which some of our authors give voice, or in the authors' voices themselves.

We use the muting metaphor to place the contributions to this volume into two groups. In the first section, "Softened Voices," are two kinds of chapters: those whose authors themselves are saying messages likely to be softened, and second, contributions about women whose voices have been softened. The research reported by the first of these types of chapters makes small but useful additions to an existing canon. They do not resist the dominant paradigm or canon of the research; rather they extend it. But in that some extensions challenge previously drawn conclusions, the findings risk being toned down or belittled if not overlooked altogether. Several chapters in this section deal with the mechanisms by which voices are muted, both directly and by teaching others to ignore all but a small segment of voices. The second section, "Silenced/Altered Voices," includes a wide variety of voices. Some tell stories or speak a woman's truth previously, or currently, muted. Voices such as these often overlap with those that have been distorted or those that large numbers of people refuse to hear or honor. These speakers in some cases express messages so distant from an existing canon they are rejected even without a hearing. In other cases, they defy legitimized ways of knowing. And in still others, the message is rejected because the messenger is not respected. We return shortly to this discussion of why voices have not been heard.

Nine chapters comprise the first section of the book. Sylvia L. Ashwell, in "Aizuchi: Suggestions for a (Relatively) New Model of Conversation Analysis," discusses the Japanese practice of *aizuchi*, called *backchanneling* by U. S. scholars. She notes its frequent use by Japanese speakers compared to English speakers and shows the importance of understanding its association with powerlessness in English (because of its association with women) because it does not have such an association in Japanese. Without such an awareness, we cannot effectively teach English speakers to speak Japanese or Japanese speakers to speak English. Ashwell's argument is an excellent example of the small addition to existing knowledge that can be made if scholars will listen to previously unheard voices, something possible only if our own customs of communication and language do not lead us to hear alternative patterns or voices as we would hear our own. In "Women and Men in Egyptian Obituaries: Language, Gender, and Identity," Mushira Eid examines changes in how women and men are identified in Egyptian obituaries over a span of 50 years from 1938 to 1988. She reports that identification of women by name has increased greatly over that period of time, although differences remain between Muslim and Christian groups in amount and type of identification. These first two chapters are overtly comparative in the sense that the writers directly compare English patterns to a different language or communication system.

Joan Kelly Hall's chapter, "The Power of Women's Voices in the Practice of Chismeando," reports listening to the voices of women in San Christóbal, Santo Domingo as they engage in *chismeando* (gossip). From the women's talk, she draws two contributions to existing knowledge. First, she notes how the women use *chismeando* to identify, enforce, and relate to the social code. Second, and importantly, she shows that the intonation patterns of the phrase-final rise and fall cannot be interpreted to have universal meanings. As with Ashwell's chapter, Hall's analysis of *chismeando* shows how hearing previously discounted (muted) voices can modify conclusions based on previous scholarship.

Three contributions in this section pay attention to one mechanism by which voices are muted, both directly and in teaching others to ignore all but a small segment of voices. One of these, "Gender/Language Subtexts as Found in Literature Anthologies: Mixed Messages, Stereotypes, Silence, Erasure," by Mary R. Harmon uncovers the gender subtexts in five widely used anthologies of U.S. literature, all with copyright dates after 1989, four after 1990. She demonstrates that as these books propose literature to be taught in high schools, women's voices are to be small, in no case to exceed one third of the pages, in most cases to include less than one in four of the authors or pages. Her work confirms the continuing validity of Russ' arguments. Paola Traverso's chapter, "I Never Told Anybody and I Desperately Need Someone to Talk to: Problem Pages for Girls in Italian Teen Magazines," reports an analysis of the advice columns in three Italian teen magazines. She found that the magazines continue to present relationships with boys and achieving appropriate femininity as important concerns for teenaged girls while ignoring most of the social issues of note during the period of the analysis. She also finds, however, that the girls themselves are not merely passive recipients of advice. Traverso shows that the message of the teen magazine to girls suggests their voices are important in attracting men and demonstrating appropriately feminine role behavior, thus subtilely saying to the girls, "You need not talk about the serious issues."

Lenora A. Timm's, "Romancing the Earth: Feminized Nature and Maternal/Erotic Metaphors in Recent Eco-Environmental Literature," presents a message itself susceptible to softening, if not silencing or distortion. She develops an unpopular thesis, arguing that we court danger with the maternal metaphors widely used for the earth, popular in eco-environmental literature, and in much feminist writing. Challenging a popular orthodoxy invites muting.

Deborah Foreman-Takano's chapter, "Hit or Myth: The Perpetration of Popular Japanese Stereotypes in Japan-published English Textbooks," is the third contribution in this section that exposes a mechanism by which voices are silenced. She introduces a group of papers bounded by geography, in that they relate to women and language in Japan. Foreman-Takano examines writing used to teach English in Japan and shows how stereotypical attitudes about both Japan and "the West" distort depictions of both in writings used to teach English in Japan. Continuing the focus on Japanese, Naoko Ogawa's, "Age, Sex, and Linguistic Judgments: Politeness and 'Femininity'" is another contribution that can extend the canon if not muted. She reports ratings of politeness and femininity or masculinity, ratings done by a wide age range of Japanese speakers. The ratings challenge previously believed scholarly and popular conclusions that politeness and femininity are not correlated in Japanese speech. Rather, Ogawa's data show, politeness is Japanese, and not correlated with femininity. It is rudeness and masculinity that correlate. In "Female-Male Inequality in Japanese Writing," Yasuko Hio examines gender stereotypes as she discusses the distorting effect of importing Chinese characters as the basis for the writing system for Japanese.

The second part of the book includes voices muted by silencing or altering. Many of these authors are women who write in their own voice and relate insights they had as they sought to hear women's voices from earlier in their own cultural history. Or they write of their insights as they made sense of their own experiences of hearing muted voices within a different and dominant culture. The first chapter in this group, "Sexism in Japanese Society: Not What We Think It Is," by Chieko Koyama, continues the geographic/language grouping of Japan/Japanese. Koyama, whose work was motivated by her effort to make sense of her encounters with sexism in the United States, writes of the women of ancient Japan, women whose voices are softened in the Japan of the 1990s, and about whom almost nothing is heard outside that country. She expresses her own hope for recovery of those ancient voices in modern Japan. The chapter, "The Identity of Kannadigas Women: Study of Kinship and Address Systems," by Susan Shear, changes geographic focus to India. Shear writes about address systems in Kannada, the language of the Kannadigas, a Dravidian people of the southern part of India. She demonstrates a treatment of women in the language and marital customs that belies widely held beliefs about India. Hence, she shows the muted voice of Kannada within India and of the failure to hear this particular voice outside the Indian subcontinent. The next contribution, "Who Speaks for North African Women in France?" by Patricia Geesey discusses the problematic distortion of North African women's voices as they are produced and reproduced in France. Her title and chapter express well the problem of muting as altered or distorted voice in groups with varying levels of influence within a culture. Who does speak for a group of women? The question is difficult and the answers are more so.

Returning geographically to North America, the next set of contributions deals with voices often completely muted. Dominique Gendrin's work, "Homeless Women's Inner Voices: Friends or Foes?" analyzes voices almost never heard and even less honored—conversations that are imagined by homeless women—and assesses the value of such conversations to the women who carry on these internal dialogues. She suggests encouraging the use of these internal, personal voices to help avoid the social isolation and desperation brought about by becoming homeless. In "Cherokee Generative Metaphors," Lisa Perry writes of the generative metaphors of the Cherokee, a group whose voices a long and conscious effort attempted not only to silence but to eliminate—an effort not yet dead with the rise of English-only movement in the United States in the 1990s. LaTasha Farmer's "Sexual Harassment and Catcalls among African Americans," notes that growing acceptance of the idea of sexual harassment has potential to distort understanding of the practice of verbal interplay among African Americans.

Toward the end of the book, we include three widely disparate chapters. Each fits the metaphor of muting in different ways. David Natharius' paper, "The Stifling of Women's Voices: Men's Messages From Men's Movement Books," examines three widely read books of the Men's Movement. Through his outlines of the arguments in these books, Natharius shows how many men mute the voices of women in the feminist movement. His analysis of the men's voices makes clear the amount of distortion in their understanding of what women are saying and how little they actually listen to women's voices. Next, we include Leilani Cook's "Magical Voices," a transcription and discussion of the words of two women whose voices are widely dismissed, muted by being ignored or disparaged. These are women of magic, a Wiccan and a Catholic faith healer; Cook describes the two women at work. Louise Gouëffic, whose words from "The Patriarchal Code Works Against the Common Good of all Individuals," open this introduction, closes the book with a chapter both academic and artistic. She summarizes her analysis of The Patriarchal Code, 10,000 words in English that she sees as supporting "man in his role as father-husband-man and son, as the basis of act, thought, and reasoning." She argues that exposing the Code will lay bare the "deep level structure of male bias or 'sexism'" found in English. The sweep of her view and unorthodoxy of her method have led many to dismiss both the argument and the arguer.

UNDERSTANDING OUR OWN VOICES

Several of these authors comment explicitly on the problems they (or their consultants) confront when crossing cultural language borders. The concerns go beyond the matter of learning a new vocabulary and the obvious rules of the grammar of a language. In learning to operate within a different language and cultural system, we need to understand our own voice. The issue here goes farther than what most of us call easily to mind when we think about our English language. Any communication system operates within a cultural system, and both include rules of thinking, talking, and communicating that native speakers know and (they might say "intuitively") do without noticing, or sometimes even knowing what they have done. These unstated patterns, of which most speakers are unaware, guide how we think communication should (must) occur; then, often without understanding these patterns, we apply rules that fit our system but not others.

Many rules of communication relate to gender and these cultural rules about gender and communication are among those least likely to be taught explicitly. As a result, gender rules, which communication almost always involves, are those most likely to be applied without conscious awareness. At the same time, the gender rules of cultures vary widely, so are potentially the source of many and various interpretations of how communication transactions should be carried out.

Because of the diversity of voices brought together in this volume, it is necessary to foreground the gender rules buried in the communication of English speakers. These patterns of English thinking reflected in the logic of our grammar and in the unstated premises on which we operate provide the frame for how we perceive what we see and hear and read and how we understand the materials in this book. For that reason, we include here a brief summary of previous work that exposes the underlying assumptions about gender that inform the perceptual schemata of English speakers. We then use the chapters in this volume to discuss how our assumptions about gender, language and communication combine to silence a wide variety of women's voices.

As English speakers, we have built a whole system of thinking on the assumption that the human species is divided into two genders, arising out of our two sexes. Gender, virtually everyone now agrees, is a social-cultural phenomenon that has to do with behaviors, values, attributes, expectations, relationships, and so on, in addition to being an identity category. However, few cultures, and certainly not English-speaking ones, have anything like a clear set of agreements about exactly what those behaviors, values, and so forth are. Thus expectations related to gender do not break clearly into "two" groups. Perhaps more problematic, however, are other assumptions about sex that we transfer to assumptions about gender: There are only two genders, no more. Female persons will develop (and exhibit) feminine genders; male persons will develop (and exhibit) masculine genders. No one individual will develop (or exhibit) more than one gender. Once achieved, a person's gender does not change; it is not influenced by relationships, situations, or passage of time. As we live our lives, these assumptions hold only for a very few people, unless gender is defined in such a way as to remove everything from the definition except one's decision that one is female or male.

For some people, none of the assumptions hold. Many people with the "wrong" chromosomes develop female gender identities and some people with no Y chromosomes develop male gender identities. Although modern surgical techniques and modern media have permitted wider awareness of such "anomalies," such inconsistencies are not new phenomena. Nor have they been created by "modern" civilization. Some cultures have legitimized gender identities that were inconsistent with external genitalia; others have attributed special status to persons who possessed biological manifestations of both sexes.

Important about the incorrectness of these assumptions is how they relate to the way women's voices are heard. To begin to unravel the complexity of the influences, a set of definitions given by Kessler and McKenna (1978) is useful. Kessler and McKenna described gender as multifaceted, distinguishing as different gender assignment (what infants are labeled at birth), gender identity (what one calls oneself), gender role, and gender attribution (what gender other people decide a person is). Gender attribution is the most useful concept. Gender attribution is something each of us does whenever we interact with others. First, we decide a person's sex, and then continually draw conclusions about that person and gender. Similarly, although less significant for this discussion, each of us constantly behaves in ways that present cues that lead others to make gender attributions about us. When one interacts with others, almost no communication can take place until we resolve the question: "Is this person female or male?" Usually the conclusion is drawn quickly, with little or no conscious thought. But it is almost always drawn, and once made, the decision then triggers numerous subsequent attributions affecting the subsequent communication.

Ordinarily, we do not focus on such "doing" of gender. We have learned patterns of interaction and repeat them without much attention until we encounter new people or new situations that require alteration in the pattern. In the doing and learning over many years, not only have we developed habitual patterns that we enact without paying attention, we also develop feelings and attitudes about gender. These feelings also operate without conscious awareness until some challenge or event calls them to the surface.

One could use the analogy of an iceberg as a useful way to conceptualize these aspects of gender. Weaver (1985) used such an analogy to describe how culture functions; doing gender is much the same way. Weaver noted that what we observe about a culture is a relatively small part of its impact, in the same way as the part of an iceberg that appears above the surface of the water is much smaller than that below the surface. The analogy can apply to gender as well. In doing gender, what we "see" (or at least pay attention to) are behaviors and language. Habitual patterns and attitudes about behaviors and language are not visible, but quite strong. And the attitudes, feelings, and judgments about patterns of gendered behavior and values powerfully affect communication.

One final concept is helpful to understand the role of gender in the creation of meaning about women and women's voices, the idea of cognitive schemata. A *cognitive schema* is a collection of organizing ideas or principles that play a major role in interpretations of subsequent perceptions and experiences. Schemata can be described as working models for how "the world is" that we develop as we learn a culture. Through life experiences, schemata can (and do) change, but schema are generally conservative. We tend to assimilate new information to fit existing schemata.

Gender schemata involve aspects of personal identity, ideas about others, ideas about interpersonal and public interaction among people, ideas about cultural roles and norms, and ideas about language and language use. One of the basic impacts of gender in communication is that our schemata about humans include the belief that they must be gendered—and each culture imposes many constraints on how that gender exists and is expressed. In other words, each culture encourages the development of particular gender schema that guide and focus behavior of people within that culture. Another way to put it is that schemata focus and frame gender into ideologies that create ways of thinking.

Bem (1993) used the metaphor of a lens to describe gender schemata. Ideas of gender, whether individuals' gender schemata or more generalized cultural ideas of gender create ways of seeing, hence the term, *lens*. Bem believes that most of us look through these lenses, hence they determine how we see the world. Importantly, we interpret the lenses as showing how things are, not as just another way of seeing. Bem argued that we need to look at the lenses, not through them, to see the impact of gender in our lives.

Bem identified three gender lenses within our gender schemata: androcentrism, gender polarization, and biological essentialism. Androcentrism, a term first used by the First Wave feminist Charlotte Perkins Gilman, is male centeredness—the equation of what is male or masculine with standard. Bem pointed out that androcentrism is not "the historically crude perception that men are inherently superior to women, but a more treacherous underpinning of that perception," one that identifies female as a sex-specific deviation from the norm and male or masculine with human (p. 2). *Androcentrism*, for example, sees women as the weaker sex and, therefore, male strength as standard. Another example: The male voice is standard leading to the interpretation that women's voices are weak or soft. Androcentric thinking assumes that life forms are male unless proven otherwise and that the way men do things is the norm. An androcentric view would not describe women's voices as standard and men as speaking loudly and intrusively.

Now, to be sure, androcentric views in U.S. culture hold a particular view of male as the standard. It is a White, Eurocentric version of male that all else is measured by the size of its deviation. Deviations from the Euro-masculine model—to be female, or Black, indeed to be any race besides White—is to be not just different, but nonstandard, deviant.

The second gender lens named by Bem (1993) is *gender polarization*. This involves the assumptions about gender identified earlier: There are two, and only two, unchanging genders; females develop and do feminine gender; males develop and do masculine gender. These assumptions create a lens because the relationship between female and male is presumed dichotomous. Gender polarization becomes the organizing principle for the social life of the culture. It is expected, not merely that females and males will differ, do different things, communicate differently, and so on, but also that the differences are dichotomous. Polarization adds to the perniciousness of androcentrism. Polarization makes being not male into the opposite of male.

A third gender lens is *biological essentialism*. One who subscribes to biological essentialism believes that the assumptions built into both of the other lenses, but especially gender polarization, are the natural and inevitable consequences of intrinsic biological givens. A biological essentialist argues that biology causes gender polarization. That researchers have devoted years of study continuing to attempt to answer questions about differences between women and men, while ignoring questions about differences among women, and among men, demonstrates the power of the biological essentialism lens. Its power is also demonstrated by the continuing efforts to demonstrate how biology causes a whole variety of human behavior, including human communication patterns. That folks, both lay and scientific, on either side of the argument, will not easily accept a conclusion that the causes of human behavior lie both in environment and biology illustrates the power of the interactive influence of two lenses, gender polarization, and biological essentialism.

A final point about the biological essentialism lens: To suggest this is a perceptual screen rather than a "fact" is in reference to gender characteristics across a culture. For any individual, biology may be to some extent deterministic. One's size, propensity to have allergies, level of activity, or any of hundreds of other characteristics may be, probably are, strongly influenced by one's biology. Even for individuals, however, the outcomes are not determined by biology. A person with genes to become large will not grow to full potential if she or he is inadequately nourished as a child. Even more so is variability exhibited across the many individuals within a culture. The biological essentialist, however, believes that biology determines gender polarization across a culture, with a resulting belief that the polar opposites of gender apply to all women and men, and if there are individuals who do not display these characteristics, they are deviants or in some way abnormal.

Bem (1993) noted only three gender lenses, but Taylor (1996) argued that in current English-speaking cultures there exists a fourth gender lens. This lens is the premise of *heterosexual essentialism*, an idea extrapolated from Rich (1976, 1980). Among the fundamental assumptions we make about gender is the expectation that females will be attracted to males and only to males; and that males will be attracted to females and only to females. The belief is that "normal" people "naturally" behave in these ways. Heterosexuality is seen as the way biology predisposed individuals, hence the essentialistic label. A construction of gender relations as essentially heterosexual is deep within our scientific, philosophical, and cultural understandings of "how things are." One outcome is our conclusion that those without the "natural" sexual attractions are deviants and abnormal. Thus, a generally shared cultural belief has been that to be homosexual, or bisexual, is to be abnormal, sick, or sinful. The assumption of heterosexual relationships undergirds virtually every one of our cultural institutions. The supremacy of this lens is being challenged, but on the whole it remains a dominant perspective.

Throughout, this discussion of the four lenses reflects an underlying principle that ties them all together. Something beyond the lenses is necessary, for example, to convert androcentrism from a description of how things are to an assertion of what should be. To convert male as standard into male as ideal requires a ranking principle. Such a ranking principle underlies the constant suggestion that to be different from a norm is deficient; that of two "opposites" one is better; that biology is "more" important than culture or environment. In each case, the "need" to rank cannot be accounted for with only the gender lenses Bem described.

An additional element is at work. We describe it as the *hierarchy principle*. The hierarchy principle is also a cognitive schema, perhaps among the most important in influencing how we construe the world to be. (A perceptive reader will note that the preceding sentence is an example of what it is saying.) The hierarchy principle pervades our thinking; one can find it in almost every idea expressed and every sentence spoken.

Hardman (1993) first articulated the hierarchy principle in relation to gender in her work on derivational thinking. Hardman described derivational thinking by showing how three postulates of

English underlie or reflect patterns of thinking.[4] By postulate, Hardman referred to a concept that is "manifested structurally across all the levels of a grammar within a culture" (p. 42). A postulate is so much a part of the grammar, it reflects (or is) a way of thinking. The postulates she named are of number, of ranking (the comparative-superlative), and of sex-based gender. The first two of these postulates do not appear to be about gender, but because the relation among the three is mutually reinforcing, they are inextricably linked, and reflect (and in turn create) a gendered way of thinking by English speakers. One could summarize the three postulates with the following trilogy: Number is important; number one is most important; number one is masculine. Significant for this discussion is the way Hardman's work illustrates the hierarchy principle and applies it to gender.

The postulate of number simply reflects that, with very few exceptions, English speakers must make decisions about number whenever they talk. To speak in English, one must know whether the subject of the sentence is singular or plural, which then determines the remainder of how one talks about that subject. The exceptions to the postulate of number are mostly unmodified imperatives ("get out," "Be careful"). But even such imperatives imply a clear sense of the second postulate, the postulate of ranking. Some rank is implied when one speaker assumes the right to give another orders or instructions. The postulate of hierarchy (ranking) reflects the English speaker's constant drive to compare in a ranking manner. All native speakers of English understand (and constantly use) the postulate of hierarchy when they apply the comparative-superlative principle ("You are wise; she is wiser; I am wisest"). We use the principle constantly.

Hardman (1993) suggested doubting readers try doing without a comparative or superlative ranking in their speech for as little as 1 hour. She reported challenging students to listen to themselves and try to avoid implementing hierarchy in their speech for just 1 day. No student whose first language is English has reported success. Illustrative is the nature versus nurture controversy previously cited. Why must it be that one is "more" influential than the other? Why can't both have influence? What matters which is the "most" influential? Also

---

[4]The work on derivational thinking came out of Hardman's (1978) work on the linguistic postulate developed to describe the underlying principles of the Jaqi languages of South America, which do not include the categories that frame derivational thinking. The basic linguistic postulates of Jaqi are data source and humanness. Clearly, the early perception of the correlation between obligatory grammatical categories and the ordinary perceptions of the speakers of any language was inspired by the work of scholars who came before, in particular, the work of Lee and her work with the Wintu (1959/1987, 1986), and also the work of Sapir (1921, 1961) and Whorf (1956).

illustrative is Hardman's suggestion that in the United States, we must talk about equality constantly if we want to have any because the structure of our language (and our thinking) is built on hierarchy.[5]

In the third postulate, Hardman (1993) supplied the key to why the hierarchy principle forms a gendered lens. The third postulate is that male, or masculine, is best. In English, feminine is derived from masculine, just as in the dominant religious traditions of English speakers, female was derived from male. Hardman used the linguistic concept of *marking* to develop this point; and the argument she made has been developed in numerous ways by many other linguists (e.g., Miller & Swift, 1976; Penelope, 1990). Male, in English, is unmarked. That means male is the standard from which differences are measured, or "marked." Until recently, and still for many, for example, the word *actor* must be marked with "ess" to denote a female actor; waiter (and many other terms) similarly. Another marking that relates to gender is that marked by "ette" to denote smaller or lesser. A *dinette*, for example, is a small table; a vinyl couch may be described as *leatherette* (unless you want to sell it!). The relation to gender is probably obvious, but some examples may be instructive. *Coquette*, for example, in English is applied to females even though the French from which it is derived (*coqueter*: to flirt; *coquette*: a beau, a flirt, a little cock) was not female-specific. For a communication-related example, take the term *suffragette* applied to the women of the 19th-century voting rights movement. They never used the term themselves. If they described themselves as other than crusaders for women's rights it was as *suffragists*. First derisively and later because to English speakers it seemed the appropriate term, they became (and the uninitiated call them yet today) suffragettes. A native speaker of English would identify a suffragist as a person (e.g., a man) who seeks suffrage. Another example is the case mentioned earlier, of man as the common term for *homo sapiens*.

An example of derivational thinking that is also grammatical, involving the three postulates, is the ranking of object and subject within a sentence, and then assigning preferred gender to these grammatical slots. Such assignment underlies our linking passivity and victimization (object status) to femininity and agentiveness (subject status) to masculinity. Thus, if anything bad befalls anyone, it is the woman's fault; if anything good or worthwhile is done, men do it.

Derivational thinking, then, the constant and mutually reinforcing use of these three grammatical structures, is the way in which we grammaticalize some of the schemata previously mentioned.

---

[5]Mizutani (1981) argued that the reverse is true for Japanese—who must talk about ranking because the basic structure is equality.

It is also why we find it so difficult to change our assumptions and ways of perceiving, even though it be our desire to do so, and why it is so difficult for us to appreciate diversity or perceive equality.

These postulates of derivational thinking demonstrate how fundamental the gender hierarchy is to English thought. Without the hierarchy principle, androcentrism and gender polarization could describe separate and equal spheres. In that the postulates make clear how strong is the impulse to hierarchy (to ranking), recognizing them demonstrates how exceptionally difficult gender equality is for those whose thought structures are built on English. English thinkers almost compulsively rank any two items seen as related. Hence, native English speakers virtually never think of female and male, or feminine and masculine as simply different. Until the English ranking postulate is at least weakened, it will take extraordinary effort and commitment on the part of any speaker of English not to see one of any pair as best, more appropriate, more valuable, more "standard." Similarly, until we look at the gender polarization lens, it will be difficult to see any difference pair as simply different, not opposite.

The hierarchy principle interacts with the other lenses in many ways. Think of a culture developed with the same postulates, but without the androcentric lens. Give it, for example, a gynocentric lens. Number would still be important; one still best; but now one would be feminine. The ranking, polarizing, and heterosexual lenses would remain. The culture would be matriarchal, but as long as the impulse to rank remains (e.g., as long as one is best), gender polarization and inequality would remain.[6]

This excursion into understanding the definitions and assumptions about gender, the gender lenses, and the hierarchy principle that infuse English thinking provides a framework for understanding the kinds of muting that have occurred with respect to women's voices. We note here that some aspects of these assumptions, perspectives, and principles appear in other cultures, particularly but not exclusively in other Indo-European languages or cultures. Each culture involves its own set of nuances. The same behavior may or may not reflect the same

---

[6]The Jaqi do not rank people by sex; women and men are equal within the culture—both human, as contrasted with the nonhuman. Equal, not identical. As Hardman explained to students and others, the common perception is that, if men are not dominant, then women are; so, if it is not a patriarchy then it has to be a matriarchy. Endless explanations that no, it is *not* a matriarchy, but rather a culture where all adult persons are *human* fall on deaf ears, or, rather, into brains that run on the rails of derivational thinking. For additional information about the Jaqi languages see Hardman (1966, 1981, 1982, 1984, 1985, 1986), and Hardman, Yapita, de Dios, and Vásquez (1988).

categories of thinking. We must take great care neither to misperceive nor fail to see structures to which we are oblivious because we categorize according to our own patterns of thinking. Especially, but not only outside of the Indo-European family, what appear to us to be similar behaviors may very well be reflecting structures quite foreign to us. Using our own patterns of thought without focusing on them can blind us to assumptions, perspectives, and principles of other cultures. This is in part what happened as colonialism denigrated the status of women in many "conquered" cultures in order to bring those cultures into line with derivational thinking.

Many of the chapters in this book demonstrate some or all of the effects of the gendered thought patterns just discussed. Perry's work on Cherokee came about specifically as she came to understand the role that derivational thinking had played in the misunderstandings that she faced on a daily basis as well as those of her culture historically. Shear's examination of Kannada kinship and address systems emerged as she learned through personal contact that what she had been told about India did not match her experiences. Koyama's discussion of popular stories that convey conventional understandings of gender, specifically women, grew out of discussions of derivational thinking with an English-speaking friend and her surprise in learning the underlying grammatical categories and perceptual schemata of English speakers and that English speakers lacked the stories of strong powerful women in influential roles that she assumed everyone knew. Farmer's study of catcalling among her African-American friends resulted from her effort to apply a dominant cultural perspective and definitions of sexual harassment to the life she lives.

Similarly, the interaction of these gendered patterns of thinking and talking have often resulted in the silencing of voices, some of whom we hope to recover in this book. Koyama and Hio, who examines Japanese ideographic writing, both work to explore traces of ancient voices within existing language and cultural patterns. Koyama's work, especially, demonstrates the danger of applying to one culture gender schema appropriate to another. Belief in and interpretation of the powerlessness of Japanese women derive in part from seeing one culture's interaction patterns through the lens of another culture. Hall's conclusions based on a devalued community are part of a specific effort to suggest that less hierarchical conception of the value of people (and thus of their speech). Both Ashwell's work on *aizuchi* and Ogawa's study of politeness and gender demonstrate gender subtexts in that they both show how people "really" talk differs from gendered expectations.

Many of the chapters show the hierarchy principle at work, combined with polarization and applied to cultural differences. A kind of "unconscious" cultural ranking is demonstrated in Foreman-Takano's examination of English textbooks; Shear's discussion of Kannada; Ashwell's look at *aizuchi;* Hall's analysis of *chismeando.* The combined effects of gender polarization and hierarchy are discussed in Gendrin's study of homeless women's self-conversations; Eid's analysis of obituaries; Traverso's look at the content of teen magazines in Italy; Natharius' report of how men in the men's movement view women. Cook's women of magic themselves demonstrate how voices are devalued in part due to gender identification and in part due to other types of hierarchy at work. Natharius' review of men's movement books especially highlights the strength of the hierarchy principle. These writers cannot conceive that female and male could both be hurt in our existing system; to improve women's status would put women above men they believe; they cannot imagine equality. If men cannot dominate women, then obviously, they think, women must dominate men. The writers reflect the strength of the polarization lens as well. Men cannot have a feminine side; they must reject it to become "real" men because to be feminine in any way means to be not masculine. The conclusion is absurd to anyone who sees the gender lenses instead of looking at the world through them.

Several of the chapters show the complexity involved in the interactions among the elements in our gender schemata and other thought patterns. Among these are Timm's analysis of the complexity and unanticipated potentials of gendered language; and Geesey's examination of how one woman is taken to speak for others even when speaking of her own experience. And although the chapters themselves do not always draw out the full potential implication of these complex interactions, many of the issues are ripe for such analysis.

In that respect, it is helpful to turn to the discourse strategies of silencing that Russ (1983) described. These include denial of agency ("She didn't really do it"); pollution of agency ("She did it, but look who she is," or "she did it but she had help"); false categorization ("She's just a children's writer"); dual standard of content ("Women's life experiences are of no interest"); anomalousness ("She's an eccentric"); and isolation ("She only wrote one"). Russ' categories actually turn out to be specific ways in which the gender schemata and derivational thinking implement their goals of establishing hierarchy and the primacy of androcentric values. It must be remembered that the hierarchy principle can be generalized beyond gender to class, race, and other categories conceived to be "less than" the ideal of White and male. So, the variation on the agency premise is "They didn't really do and if they did it doesn't count because . . . (they are no good people, the work is 'just' a . . . , their lives are of no interest, they're weird, and there's only one of them)" irrespective of any relevance of these statements to actual factual truth.

Many of the chapters illustrate one or more of Russ' principles at work. For example, *chismeando* is gossip, by women, and therefore is not important. Not to be listened to seriously, it would rarely be thought of as contributing to linguistic or communication theory. *Aizuchi*, considered a practice of the Japanese (and thought wrongly of referring to Japanese women primarily), is considered in the United States as a polite behavior, or a feminine behavior; therefore, it is of no interest, along with the people perceived to do it. Although now with the advent of Japan as an economic superpower the discounting of Japanese men is difficult, it gets done in another way, in attributions of insincerity and opaqueness—pollution of agency. Ogawa's examination of the associations with politeness sheds light on another side of the process and in so doing illustrates the interactions among the gender lenses. Politeness has been associated with femininity and with women, even by scholars who should know better, and labeled as *weakness behavior*.[7] Androcentrism and hierarchy have associated two devalued concepts and led us to ignore other associations, in this case rudeness and masculinity. The complexity of the associations of gendered language is also exposed in Timm's discussion of the feminine metaphors in eco-environmentalism, which also illustrates pollution of agency and false categorization.

Harmon's analysis of anthologies of literature clearly demonstrates Russ' categories at work, and is an update of a portion of Russ' work, showing that the categories discussed in 1983 were still valid in 1994. If "she" wrote it, the literature cannot be as important or good as that written by men. Women's writing warrants having only short pieces or few pieces included. The same analysis applies to the dismissal of foreign or lower class voices. If "they" do it, it can't be worthwhile.

Many of the voices of the authors presented here are not the traditional voices found in a "scholarly" book. We have some concern that Russ' categories, applied to women or class-based, might lead to the dismissal of some of the contributions to this book: a pollution of agency (the homeless or women of magic), a false categorization (gossip or immigrants or non-Whites or metaphors of mother earth), a double standard of content (teen aged girls or Gouëffic's creative philology or the lives of immigrants or natives); or anomalousness (again, women of magic or creative philology or Kabyle women in France). Some of the chapters deal with instances in which "she didn't do it." That would

---

[7]The Spanish have a saying, *Lo cortés no quita lo valiente* (Courtesy does not negate the presence of valor), which reflects as it denies this association. It is used to encourage courtesy even when anger is appropriate.

appear to be the case of Egyptian obituaries, where the lives led would appear to be those of the men, not the women themselves. This book itself is at risk of being dismissed because "there is only one of it."

We are convinced, however, that appreciation of diversity and the richness of many different patterns of communicating depends on our ability to perceive value across differing styles of voice. To be able to do that, to accept widely varying voices as having something to contribute to our understanding of the human condition, we must make the effort and commitment necessary to hear outside the postulates of our derivational thinking, to go beyond the boundaries of our own gendered thinking. We must learn to hear the voices of women and the voices of other cultures as serious, as standard, as also part of the norm of humankind.

The ambition of the conference of *Our Own and Others' Voices* was to contribute toward that dream. The intent of *Hearing Many Voices* is the same. We offer here a diversity of voices that may be heard as standard, normal parts of the intricately woven human quilt. We hope our readers will hear the voices in that manner.

REFERENCES

Ardener, E. (1975). The "problem" revisited. In S. Ardener (Ed.), *Perceiving women* (pp. 19-27). London: Malaby Press.

Ardener, S. (Ed.). (1975). *Perceiving women*. London: Malaby Press.

Bellah, R. N., Madsen, R., Sullivan, W. M., Sidler, A., & Tipton, S. M. (1985). *Habits of the heart: Individualism and commitment in American life*. New York: Harper & Row.

Bem, S. L. (1993). *The lenses of gender: Transforming the debate on sexual inequality*. New Haven, CT: Yale University Press.

Brantenberg, G. (1985). *Egalia's daughters*. Seattle: Seal Press.

Davis, A. Y. (1981). *Women race & class*. New York: Vintage Books.

Elgin, S. H. (1984). *Native tongue*. New York: Daw Books.

Elgin, S. H. (1987). *The Judas rose*. New York: Daw Books.

Elgin, S. H. (1994). *Earthsong*. New York: Daw Books.

Gage, M. J. (1980). *Woman, church & state* (S. R. Wagner, ed.). Watertown, MA: Persephone Press. (Original work published 1893)

Hardman, M. J. (1966). *Jaqaru: Outline of phonological and morphological structure*. The Hague: Mouton.

Hardman, M. J. (1978). Andean ethnography: The role of language structure in observer bias. *Semiotica, 71*(3/4), 339-372.

Hardman, M. J. (Ed.). (1981). *The Aymara language in its social and cultural context* (University of Florida Social Sciences Monograph No. 67). Gainesville: University Presses of Florida.

Hardman, M. J. (1982). The mutual influences of Spanish and the Andean languages. *Word, 33*(1/2), 71-77.

Hardman, M. J. (1984, Winter). Gentiles in Jaqi folktales—An example of contact literature. *Anthropological Linguistics,* 367-375.

Hardman, M. J. (1985). The imperial languages of the Andes. In N. Wolfson & J. Manes (Eds.), *Language of inequality* (pp 183-193). University Park: University of Pennsylvania.

Hardman, M. J. (1986). Data source marking in the Jaqi languages. In W. Chafe & J. Nichols (Eds.), *Evidentiality: The linguistic coding of epistemology* (pp. 113-136). Norwood, NJ: Ablex.

Hardman, M. J. (1993). Gender through the levels. *Women and Language, 16*(2), 42-49.

Hardman, M. J. (1994). "And if we lose our name, then what about our land?" or, What price development? In L. H. Turner & H. M. Sterk (Eds.), *Differences that make a difference: Examining the assumptions in gender research* (pp. 151-162). Westport & London: Bergin & Garvey.

Hardman, M. J., Yapita M., de Dios, J., & Vasquez, J., with Martin–Barber, L., Briggs, L. T., & England, N. (1988). *Compendio de la estructural fonológica y morfológica de la lengua Aymara.* La Paz: Editorial ILCA (Instituto de Lenguaje y Cultura Aymara), Gramma Impresión.

Hill, A. O. (1986). *Mother tongue, father time: A decade of linguistic revolt.* Bloomington: Indiana University Press.

hooks, b. (1981). *Ain't I a woman: Black women and feminism.* Boston: South End Press.

Hull, G. T., Scott, P. B., & Smith, B. (Eds.). (1982). *All the women are white, all the blacks are men, but some of us are brave.* New York: The Feminist Press, Columbia University.

Kessler, S. J., & McKenna, W. (1978). *Gender: An ethnomethodological approach.* Chicago: University of Chicago Press.

Kramaerae, C. (1974). Women's speech: Separate but unequal? *The Quarterly Journal of Speech, 60,* 14-24.

Kramaerae, C. (1981). *Women and men speaking.* Rowley, MA: Newbury House.

Lee, D. (1987). *Freedom and culture.* Prospect Heights, IL: Waveland Press. (Original work published 1959)

Lee, D. (1986). *Valuing the self: What we can learn from other cultures.* Prospect Heights, IL: Waveland Press. (Original work published 1976)

Miller, C., & Swift, K. (1976). *Words and women: New language in new times.* Garden City, NY: Anchor Books.

Mizutani, O. (1981). *Japanese: The spoken language in Japanese life* (J. Ashby, Trans.). Tokyo: The Japan Times Ltd.

Penelope, J. (1990). *Speaking freely: Unlearning the lies of the fathers' tongues.* New York: Pergamon Press.

Rich, A. (1976). *Of woman born: Motherhood as experience and institution.* New York: Norton.

Rich, A. (1980). Compulsory heterosexuality and lesbian existence. *Signs: Journal of Women in Culture and Society, 5*(4), 631-660.

Russ. J. (1983). *How to suppress a woman's writing.* Austin: University of Texas Press.

Sapir, E. (1961). *Selected writings on language, culture and personality* (D. Mandelbaum, ed.). Berkeley: University of California Press.

Sapir, E. (1921). *Language.* New York: Harcourt, Brace & World.

Spender, D. (1980). *Man made language.* London: Routledge & Kegan Paul.

Taylor, A. (1996, May). *A proposal for a theory of gender in communication.* Paper presented at the annual convention of the Eastern Communication Association, New York City.

Tickner, A. J. (1992). *Gender and international relations: Feminist perspectives on achieving global security.* New York: University of Columbia Press.

Wagner, S. R. (1980). Introduction. In M. J. Gage (Ed.), *Woman, church & state* (pp. xv-xxxix). Watertown, MA: Persephone Press.

Washington, M. H. (1990). Foreword. In Z. N. Hurston, *Their eyes were watching god* (pp. vii-xiv). New York: Harper & Row.

Weaver, G. (1985). *Cultures in contact* [Video] (B. Broome, Producer). Fairfax, VA: George Mason University.

Whorf, B. L. (1956). *Language, thought and reality.* Cambridge: MIT Press.

LANGUAGE NOTES

Japanese is a language spoken by approximately 122 million people in Japan, and by immigrants living in the United States, Brazil, and other countries. It is not clearly related to any other language, but some linguists have considered it to be a part of the Altaic language family, whereas others relate it to the Korean language. There are several major dialect differences, with the southern dialects of the Ryukyu Islands (south of the island of Kyushu) and the Tokyo dialect (where standard Japanese comes from) forming the biggest differences. Major borrowings from other languages come from Chinese and English.

Kabyle is one of the Berber languages spoken by some 12 million people in the area known as the Maghreb or Maghrib, which is the area of north Africa including Tunisia, Algeria, and Morocco. People from this area are known as the Maghribi. Berber is a Semitic language of the eastern Sudanic family. It is not Arabic and only very distantly related; offense is taken at any attempt to link the two.

Cherokee is the southernmost language of the Iroquoian family of languages. Originally spoken in the area that is today North Carolina, most of the Cherokees were removed to Oklahoma in the Trail of Tears in the 19th century. During the 19th century, a man by the name of Sequoya developed a syllabary for writing Cherokee. The California redwoods were named in honor of this man. Today, Cherokee children are learning or relearning Cherokee in Cherokee classrooms and are again writing with the Cherokee alphabet. There are more than 10,000 speakers of Cherokee today, with only one tenth of them living in the ancestral area. The data presented here come from the eastern branch of the Cherokee.

Arabic is spoken by some 150 million people worldwide. The Egyptian variety is spoken by about 53 million people. Arabic is a Semitic language, forming a branch in and of itself, with many varieties within the language itself. The Koranic, classical or literary, Arabic exists in a diglossic relationship with the vernaculars; that is, Arabic speakers learn the latter at home and in school learn the former.

Black English, also known as Black English Vernacular (BEV) or Afro-American Vernacular English (AAVE), or, more recently, Ebonics, is a variety of English spoken by many millions of people, mostly Black, primarily in the United States. Whether this is a dialect of the English language or one language in the English family of languages has been, and is, a topic of much discussion. Black English is, in part, a creole from slave times also much influenced by southern White English.

Spanish is a Romance language descending from Latin, and is spoken by about 270 million people world wide and is currently the fastest growing minority language in the United States. The Dominican variety of Spanish is spoken by some 7 million people. Spanish was the first European language to be recognized as a language, and to be described in a grammar. The first recognition of Spanish occurred about one millennium ago; the first grammar was in 1492.

Kannada is a Dravidian language spoken by some 26 million people in southwest India in the State of Karnataka. It is not related to the Indic (e.g., Hindi) languages of northern India. Kannada has its own alphabet; inscriptions date from the sixth century and there is a literary tradition dating from the ninth.

Italian is a Romance language descending from Latin, and is spoken by some 5 million people in Italy. It is also spoken in Switzerland, the Vatican, and San Marino and is a major immigrant language in the United States, Australia, Canada, Brazil, Argentina, and to some extent Africa.

Part One

SOFTENED VOICES

1

AIZUCHI:
SOME SUGGESTIONS FOR A
(RELATIVELY) NEW MODEL OF
CONVERSATION ANALYSIS

SYLVIA L. ASHWELL

Day-to-day conversation is the most prevalent form of our communication with one another. The backbone of conversation is the interaction of the participants, that complex interplay of speech and silence in which there would be no understanding otherwise. One part of this interaction is a device called *backchanneling*, a term coined by Yngve (1970). A backchannel is a short verbal or nonverbal signal inserted by the listener when the speaker offers a space in the flow of talk without necessarily giving up that talk. Backchanneling is mainly a supportive device, but can also be used to show interest, get a response, or receive clarification. Examples include expressions like "mm-hmm," "uh-huh," "yeah," and also nonverbal signals, such as head nods and eye gaze. These backchannels usually occur at pauses in the speech flow, which sometimes can be signaled by tag questions such as: "Isn't that so?" or "Right?" (Marche & Peterson, 1993).

Backchannels, even though seemingly insignificant, are important components of conversation. The name itself suggests that *backchannels* are not important because they are not part of the "main" channel of communication but are part of the back, or less important, channel (Yngve, 1970). I prefer to use the term *aizuchi*, borrowed from the Japanese. *Aizuchi* means "hammering together," a more apt metaphor for the real meaning of conversation. Most Japanese, when asked, know about *aizuchi*. *Aizuchi* is important to the Japanese. Looking at *aizuchi* gives clues into the organization of Japanese conversation. My focus, however, is on how the structure of Japanese society informs how the Japanese people conduct conversation, on understanding contrasting English and Japanese uses of the phenomenon of *aizuchi*. Finally, I suggest a way of studying conversation in general that includes supportive devices like *aizuchi*, and a practical use for recognizing the cultural differences in using this specific conversational device (Mizutani, 1981).

DEFINITION OF *AIZUCHI*

In Japanese, *aizuchi* is found in such expressions as *un* ("yeah"), *hai* ("yes"), and *soo* ("is that right?") The use of *aizuchi* is signaled by certain syntactic markers, which roughly translate into English tag questions; some examples include *ne*, *sa*, and *yo*. These markers, which happen at the end of clauses, are followed by a short pause, which cues the listener to supply the appropriate *aizuchi*. These clauses are defined by Maynard (1989) as pause-bounded phrasal units (PPUs). PPUs can be anything from full grammatical sentences (with a subject, object, and verb) to a noun or verb phrase alone. *Aizuchi* typically occurs after PPUs, but can also occur during them. *Aizuchi* are mainly used during a topic change in the conversation and when agreement is sought. This is a fairly frequent conversational device in Japanese; in one study, there was a 35-minute conversation in Japanese in which more than 600 examples of *aizuchi* were found. What does the use of *aizuchi* in Japanese say about the Japanese language on the whole? For this, we need to look at the Japanese language more closely.

THE JAPANESE LANGUAGE AND THE *SOTO/UCHI* DISTINCTION

The main component in the Japanese grammatical system is the *soto/uchi* (outgroup/ingroup) distinction (Mizutani, 1981; Wetzel, 1994). Much of what is said in Japanese is determined by the social position and age of the person one is addressing. Members of one's *soto* group include those who are higher in social and economic position than oneself, such as employers, high government officials, and educators. High social position also includes people of advanced age; however, some aged individuals are part of one's *uchi* (literally, "home") group (e.g., parents, grandparents). Other members of one's *uchi* include family members, close friends, and acquaintances. If one is meeting another person for the first time, that person is assumed to be *soto* and treated respectfully. The boundaries between *uchi* and *soto* are fluid, and can change with increased familiarity to another person. But the *soto/uchi* distinction is never ignored; its focus on the addressees and the inherent respect due them form the cornerstone of everyday conversation. (Wetzel, 1990)

The honorific system in Japanese for both nouns and verbs attest to this. For example, the verb "to exist" takes three forms. The most respectful form, the *sonkeigo* form, is *irasharu*. This form is used when addressing people who belong to the *soto* group and, as suggested in the previous sentence, is very respectful; the neutral form, *iru*, with members of the *uchi* group; and *kenjoogo*, or humble, form, *mairu*, when referring to oneself in the presence of members of the *soto* group and esteemed members of the *uchi* group. All Japanese verbs have these three forms. Also, nouns that are attributable to a person of high social standing or advanced age receive an honorific prefix, *o-* (native Japanese words) or *go-* (words borrowed from the Chinese). For example, *o-hon no sensei* would translate literally as "the (honored) book of the professor." The word *sensei* ("teacher") illustrates the next example of honorifics: the honorific suffixes. Professors, elementary and secondary school teachers, doctors, and other persons of authority are called by last name plus *sensei* (e.g., Ashwell-*sensei*). Others that are respected in Japanese society receive the suffixes *-san* (less formal) or *-sama* (more formal). These examples from the Japanese grammatical system illustrate the importance of the *soto/uchi* distinction (Mizutani, 1981).

The use of kinship terms and other terms of address also keep the listener in mind. Figure 1.1 (adapted from Suzuki, 1978) shows the different terms of address that are a part of a Japanese person's social and personal relationships.

As the addressee changes, so do the terms of address. This is not unusual in itself; more unusual is that kinship terms can be quite fluid in Japanese. For example, one's mother is grandmother to one's children;

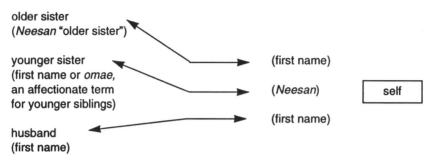

older sister
(*Neesan* "older sister")

younger sister
(first name or *omae*,
an affectionate term
for younger siblings)

husband
(first name)

(first name)

(*Neesan*)

(first name)

self

Figure 1.1. Terms of address for social and personal relationships

when one is talking with her children, one fits the children's frame of reference into her mind, and calls her own mother "grandmother." The mother starts calling her mother "grandmother" even when the children are not around. This can be true of other relatives as well (Suzuki, 1978). What becomes central to a native Japanese speaker is maintaining the relationships that one has with other people. One does this by taking the listener's frame of reference and making it her own. One tries to anticipate another's needs and wants without imposing on the other. This desire to attend to another is an integral part of the *soto/uchi* distinction. Soto/uchi depends on familiarity of, or when familiarity cannot be achieved, solicitude of the other. I explore how *aizuchi* fits into soto/uchi in the next section.

AIZUCHI AND THE *SOTO/UCHI* DISTINCTION

As noted previously, Japanese speakers use *aizuchi* (previously mentioned as backchanneling) many times in conversation. In one study comparing Japanese and English-speaking styles, Japanese used *aizuchi* three times more than did native English language users (White, 1989). Both native Japanese and native English language users carry on conversations everyday, in the workplace, with friends, and at home with family. *Aizuchi* is found in both languages. Why, then, such a marked difference in usage? The answer lies in the *soto/uchi* distinction.

A major component of *soto/uchi* is taking the listener's needs into account. *Aizuchi*, showing support in conversation, does this. By confirming what was said, the speaker knows the listener is actually listening, and the listener helps the speaker continue her talk. *Aizuchi* also shows how collaborative communication really is—how two (or more) must work together in order for communication to go smoothly. Both the speaker and listener are aware of the "hammering together" (the literal meaning of *aizuchi*) each is doing to make the conversation flow smoothly (Miller, 1991).

How does *aizuchi* fit into *soto/uchi*? Actually, a native Japanese language user uses more *aizuchi* with a member of the soto as opposed to the uchi group. Because *soto* members are typically one's superiors, and the aim in Japanese conversation is smooth relations with each other, one would supply as much *aizuchi* as possible to accomplish this end. In Yamada's (1992) study of U.S. and Japanese business discourse, he noticed that Japanese offer more *aizuchi* than the Americans in both the Japanese and English language. Again, because Japanese view Westerners and other foreigners as *soto*, Japanese would use *aizuchi* to ensure the conversation's steady and easy flow. *Aizuchi* provides a way for listeners in a conversation to interact and help out. In Japanese, it is indispensable; actually, in any language, it is absolutely necessary as well. Ask any Japanese speaker about *aizuchi*, and he or she knows what it is, but ask any English speaker about backchanneling (*aizuchi* in English) and you will get a blank stare. Most conversation analysis is done in English, why hasn't *aizuchi* been given its due?

PERCEPTIONS OF *AIZUCHI* BY NATIVE ENGLISH SPEAKERS

How is *aizuchi* viewed in English? Boxer (1993) showed that native English speakers find Japanese speakers' use of *aizuchi* in English to be excessive. As a consequence, the native speakers' perceptions of the Japanese as a whole were negative: The Japanese could offer no critical insights or comments of their own to the conversation; all the Japanese want to do is agree. This common complaint of the English of Japanese speakers carries over into more general perceptions of the Japanese— they are automatons doing what someone tells them to do; they have no originality; they cannot be independent thinkers. In other words, they are weak and have very little power in their lives to change anything. Because we stress the role of the individual in the United States, it is easy to see how a society that stresses the other can be seen as powerless. However, as Wetzel (1990) pointed out, this difference does not suggest differing degrees of power but differing definitions of power. Power is defined in Japan as coming from interactions with others and not from a person. *Aizuchi* is the center of these interactions; therefore, *aizuchi*, far from being weak and insignificant, actually is a very powerful device (Wetzel, 1990).

Another way of looking at *aizuchi* in English is as a device associated with women. Most English speakers see the supportive role played by *aizuchi* as a woman's role. Showing support or rapport is something associated with women in general, so it would seem natural that women would use more *aizuchi* than men (Tannen, 1990; Maltz & Borker, 1982, cited in Yamada, 1992). Analysis of work in conversational analysis, however, shows little difference in frequency of use of *aizuchi* in same-gender conversations in English for both females and males (Marche & Peterson, 1993). Also, in mixed-gender conversations, females and males used about the same number of *aizuchi*. Differences found in *aizuchi* use are from types, not frequency, of *aizuchi* use. Females tend to use *aizuchi* more as a support device, whereas males use it more for confirmation purposes. In any case, the differences in type are not large. This shows that although *aizuchi* is seen as feminine (and all the characteristics we associate with that), our use of *aizuchi* in English shows that it is a vital conversational device that is not gender-specific. Due to preconceptions they bring to the situation, however, English speakers tend to see the Japanese as somehow "feminine." Given the further associations of ideas of feminine, Japanese speech may also be seen as powerless. Such associations also give a sense of insignificance to *aizuchi*. Although certainly this is not the full explanation why *aizuchi* is not treated with importance, linking *aizuchi* with the "feminine" in English is at least part of the explanation. Also, English speakers are not used to the massive amount of *aizuchi* that Japanese speakers give; in their search for an explanation, may find that *aizuchi* is a symbol of powerlessness by its frequent use. An association by English speakers to "femininity" and cultural misunderstanding of *aizuchi* define the relative marginalization of this conversation device.[1]

A (RELATIVELY) NEW MODEL FOR CONVERSATION

What does this mean for the way we look at conversation? For one thing, we need to expand our view of conversation. The role of the listener or listeners needs to be fully included if we wish to know how conversation really works. This would mean examining *aizuchi* and its functions and uses, as well as other listener-support devices. This would also mean changing the meaning of "listener" and "speaker" as English speakers know it. This would be accomplished by studying other

---

[1]For an explanation of femininity and powerlessness, see Wetzel (1990) and Fishman (1978); for an illustration of marginalizing *aizuchi* and other supportive features of conversation, see Yngve (1970).

cultures and languages that have a different model for conversation than English speakers have. Examining the Japanese language is a start, but of course other languages should be studied as well. Conversation analysts should know another language well enough to get an understanding of the way things are done in that language, so they can be better informed in their work; this includes study of the nonverbal as well as verbal aspects of language. Some work has been done on the listener's role in conversation by communication researchers outside linguistics. Now it is time for linguists to give their attention to this topic. I particularly beseech native English-speaking linguists to do this; the "monolingual" approach to language studies in general is fast becoming too narrow a focus.

Why do I say a "relatively new approach"? Work done since the 1970s has seen a significant increase in examining the listener's role in conversation (Miller, 1991; Schegloff, 1982). What has been missing, however, is awareness of how much our perceptions of how people talk (i.e., our expectations based on our own rules of speech) affect our study of conversation. Boxer's (1993) study of native English speakers' perceptions of *aizuchi* is a good starting point, but a connection needs to be made between perceptions of speaking and overall perception of another culture (this includes gender as well). Both are deeply connected because the only way our perceptions can be made known is through language. Therefore, our negative perceptions of Japanese conversational style may very well inhibit us as a society from truly understanding not only these conversational styles but the Japanese people as well. To recognize these gender associations, and the associated perceptions of what is appropriate for different people to say under what circumstances, is important in teaching English to the Japanese and Japanese to the English. For language studies, it also means that we cannot come to a complete awareness of what language is until we can recognize the contributions other languages can bring us. This can be done by knowing what our perceptions of our own and the other culture are, and moving beyond them.

ACKNOWLEDGMENTS

I thank M.J. Hardman and Anita Taylor for their invaluable help in editing this chapter. Thanks also go to Diana Boxer and Ann Wehmeyer for providing sources that proved essential.

REFERENCES

Boxer, D. (1993). Complaints as positive strategies: What the learner needs to know. *TESOL Quarterly, 27*(2), 277-299.

Fishman, P. (1978). Interaction: The work women do. *Social Problems, 25,* 397-406.

Marche, T., & Peterson, C. (1993). On the gender differential use of listener responsiveness. *Sex Roles: A Journal of Research, 29*(11/12), 795-817.

Maltz, D., & Borker, R. (1982). A cultural approach to male-female miscommunication. In J. Gumperz (Ed.), *Language and social identity* (pp. 196-216). Cambridge: Cambridge University Press.

Maynard, S. (1989). *Japanese conversation: Self-contextualization through structure and interactional management.* Norwood, NJ: Ablex.

Miller, L. (1991). Verbal listening behavior in conversations between Japanese and Americans. In J. Blommaert & J. Verschueren (Eds.), *The pragmatics of intercultural and international communication* (pp. 111-130). Amsterdam: John Benjamins.

Mizutani, O. (1981). *Japanese: The spoken language in Japanese life* (J. Ashby, Trans.). Tokyo: Japan Times Ltd.

Schegloff, E. (1982). Discourse as an interactional achievement: Some uses of "uh-huh" and other things that come between sentences. In D. Tannen (Ed.), *Georgetown Round Table on languages and linguistics, analyzing discourse: Text and talk* (pp. 71-93). Washington, DC: Georgetown University Press.

Suzuki, T. (1978). *Words in context* (A. Miura, Trans.). Tokyo: Kodansha International Ltd.

Tannen, D. (1990). *You just don't understand: Women and men in conversation.* New York: Ballantine Books.

Wetzel, P. (1990). Are "powerless" communication strategies the Japanese norm? In S. Ide & N. McGloin (Eds.), *Aspects of Japanese women's language* (pp. 115-128). Tokyo: Kurosio Publishers.

Wetzel, P. (1994). A moveable self: The linguistic indexing of uchi and soto. In J. Bachnik & C. Quinn Jr. (Eds.), *Situated meaning* (pp. 73-87). Princeton, NJ: Princeton University Press.

White, S. (1989). Backchannels across cultures: A study of Americans and Japanese. *Language in Society, 18,* 59-76.

Yamada, H. (1992). *American and Japanese business discourse: A comparison of interactional styles.* Norwood, NJ: Ablex.

Yngve, V. (1970). On getting a word in edgewise. *Papers from the Sixth Regional Meeting of the Chicago Linguistic Society,* 567-577.

2

WOMEN AND MEN
IN EGYPTIAN OBITUARIES:
LANGUAGE, GENDER, AND IDENTITY

MUSHIRA EID

For most of us, a name is not just a tag or a label. It is a symbol which stands for the unique combination of characteristics and attributes that defines us as an individual. It is the closest thing that we have to a shorthand for the self-concept.
　　—Smith (1985, p. 38)

A name is so closely identified with the thing itself that *not to have a name is not to exist*.
　　—Guillaume (1938, cited in Adler, 1978, p. 98; emphasis added)

It should be self-evident—but it is not always so—that names and other descriptors of the self and others have a strong effect on people's perception of themselves and of each other. The quotes from Smith and Guillaume are only a sample of many more that can be cited as expressions of the strong relation that binds names or naming with identity.

41

But if names are indeed important in the identification of people, we would expect them to be always used. And by implication, a systematic pattern of not using names in the identification of certain people, if found, should constitute an interesting case study. Such a pattern can indeed be found in the identification of people, both deceased and survivors, in the obituary pages. Its presence, as I argued elsewhere (Eid, 1994a, 1994b), raises important questions as to the significance of identifying people with/without names and the social meaning that lies behind such linguistic choices.

If names are so important, as the quotes presented here would lead us to believe, then how can people be identified without their names, and why? The answer to the first question, as the following obituaries show, is easy: one person (A) is identified in relation to another (B) in such a way that only B's name is mentioned, thus A is identified but without a name.[1]

> Obituary 1: Passed away *Mr.* Darwish Mursi, president of the civil sector of the Asiut national court; **father** of Sayed, a student at the School of Law, Hasan, at the vocational [school], and his brother Sadiq Mursi, at the Credit Bank in Minya, and the wife of sheikh Abdel Baqi Seif at Mallawi; **maternal uncle** of Sayed Abdel Baqi at the School of Law; **relative** and **in-law** of the Dakir and Seif families. Mourning ceremonies [to be held] at Mallawi. [OB#53; 3/17/1948]

> Obituary 2: Passed into God's mercy yesterday a generous and devout lady, **mother** of the honorable Ahmad Fouad, Chief Prosecutor of Mansura; **sister** of the late *Amiralay* Mohammed *bey* Abdel Aziz; **mother-in-law** of *Bekbashi* Tawfiq Lutfi; **paternal aunt** of *Qaimmaqam* Mohammed *bek* Aziz, inspector at Misr [Cairo] Police, and Ahmad Abdel Aziz, officer in the Armed Forces; **grandmother** of the wife of Ahmad Munir in the Plants Department; **grandmother** of Abdel Aziz Tawfiq in Paris, Salih Fouad in the Law School, and Kamal el-Din Munir in the Military Academy; **maternal aunt** of the wife of Salah Eldin Eldumyati in the Italian Bank . . . [OB#37; 3/9/38][2]

---

[1]In the translation, I have tried to retain the flow of the Arabic obituary as much as possible, which at times leads to slightly awkward English as, for example, the retention of the Arabic verb first in the first obituary. To make it easier for the reader to follow the obituary texts, titles are placed in italics and relational terms in bold.

[2]In obituary 1, I used "Mr." for Arabic *ustath*, an honorific term of address used with intellectuals (lawyers, journalists, officials, writers, and poets), and in obituary 2, "the honorable" for *Hadrit*. I have also retained the Arabic military ranks for which I give equivalents here as they are given in *The Hans Wehr Dictionary of Modern Written Arabic: Amiralay*, "Colonel," *Bekbashi*, "Major," and *Qaimmaqam*, "Lieutenant Colonel."

One style of obituaries, illustrated by the two obituaries starts with a mention of the deceased through the sentence "Passed into God's mercy . . ." (or a variant thereof) followed by a list of her or his survivors and ends with information on the time and place of the funeral and other mourning ceremonies. In Obituary 1, the deceased is represented with his name (first and last "Darwish Mursi"), as well as his title ("Mr.") and occupation (president of civil sector . . .). A list of survivors follows, whereby the deceased is identified in relation to them: He is father of Sayed, and so on. Obituary 2 follows the same format, the one difference being that the name of the deceased is avoided: She is only identified as the mother of Ahmad Fouad. Her son's name is mentioned, and so is his job; he is even introduced with an honorific term of address ("the honorable"). We don't know her name; all we know about her is that she was "a generous and devout lady."

Name avoidance is used in both obituaries, but not with both deceased. In Obituary 2, it applies not only to the deceased but also to her survivors: daughter, granddaughter, and niece. To mention her daughter, the deceased is identified as "mother-in-law of *Bekbashi* Tawfiq Lutfi" (translation: mother of the wife of T. L.). Likewise, her granddaughter is listed as "the wife Ahmad Munir" and her niece as "the wife of Salah Eldin Eldumyati." Thus, all surviving females are identified through their husbands, and the deceased through her son. In Obituary 1, an obituary of a male, name avoidance is also used but only in reference to a female survivor, specifically, in identifying the daughter of the deceased as "the wife of sheikh Abdel Baqi Seif."

So although in principle any person (female or male) can be identified without a name, you may have noted in these two obituaries that it is only women that are identified without their names, not men. One of the purposes of this research is to establish the gender basis of this variation. I focus on the relation between name avoidance and women's representation in the obituaries, as well as the change that takes place over time. Name avoidance is attributed, among other things, to women's lack of public identity—itself attributed to male control over the public domain (e.g., education, economy, space) and the power associated with it, to the exclusion of women. The change in female identification takes place as women acquire education, jobs, and other public identities independent of family and home. As women begin to share resources originally reserved for men, they also get to share the linguistic resources as well. Hence, the analysis I provide supports the position that people identified without names are in some sense hidden, or nonexistent, relative to a certain domain, and that linguistic choices, like sociocultural or political choices, not only reflect the context in which they are made but also serve to reproduce or change it.

It would follow that change will be most evident when women join the workforce and participate in the sociopolitical and other public events of their community. For Egypt, I expect the 1960s was the turning point, for it was then that Egyptian women of all socioeconomic backgrounds entered the universities and the job market in large numbers, partly as a reaction to economic policies adopted by the government. (See the quotes cited from Hooglund, 1991, in the following section for some specifics.) I also expect this change to be reflected linguistically in the obituaries through the use of names, titles, and other forms of reference.

In this chapter, I report on some of the results I have obtained so far in this research; some of these findings have been discussed in more detail in Eid (1994a, 1994b). I focus on names as indicators of gender identity in the obituaries and, toward the end of the chapter, I briefly discuss the use of titles. The project as a whole is a cross-linguistic cross-cultural research on language, gender, and identity, based on a quantitative, content analysis of obituaries. It deals with three language situations: Arabic (in Egypt), Persian (in Iran), and English (in the United States), but here I only report on findings from the analysis of the Arabic obituaries. The research covers a period of 50 years, from 1938 to 1988, with data collected at 10-year intervals (1938, 1948, etc.) from one major newspaper in each country: *Al-Ahram* (Egypt), *Ittilalat* (Iran), and *The New York Times* (United States). The Arabic database consists of 1,337 obituaries; the English and Persian are comparable in size.

I begin with a brief discussion of gender inequality as revealed through the obituaries.

GENDER INEQUALITY: NAME AVOIDANCE

Previously (Eid, 1994a), I presented evidence that women in the 1938 Arabic obituaries were denied equal access to the obituary pages. Women's identity was suppressed, hidden or made invisible, whereas men's was never questioned. My analysis of the 1938 obituaries identified a number of strategies, including name avoidance, which were employed by families writing obituaries for their deceased to hide women from this public domain. These strategies serve to create a bias toward the identification, perhaps even glorification, of the male sex. But they also created the impression that this must have been a society without women, or perhaps one in which women rarely died.

A few figures illustrate the discrepancy in the representation of the sexes. First, the ratio of female to male obituaries was biased toward men (38% to 62%) suggesting that in 1938 Egyptian families tended to write obituaries for their deceased men more than they did for their deceased women. The Arabic obituaries, by comparison to their English and Persian counterparts, appeared to be more biased in this respect than the English but less so than the Persian. The English obituaries showed an almost even split for 1938 (slightly favorable to women) with 121 female to 119 male obituaries (a 50.5% to 49.5% female-male representation). Although this even split was not maintained through the years, the overall ratio was reasonably close with a 47% to 53% female-male representation. In the case of Persian, the earliest that can be compared with is 1948 where the distribution of female to male obituaries was 43% to 57%, and the overall distribution was 38% to 62%. On the basis of overall distribution, however, English came out as least biased (47% to 53%), Persian as most (38% to 62%), and Arabic as in between (41% to 59%).

A similar, if not worse, bias was found among the survivors in the 1938 Arabic obituaries. Only 30% of the obituaries mentioned female survivors—the remaining 70% of the families who chose to write obituaries for their deceased must either have had no female family members (which is highly unlikely), or they must have chosen not to mention them (which is much more likely). Worse yet, only 7 of the 148 (4.7%) obituaries obtained for that year mentioned a female survivor by name. Worst of all, however, were the statistics on gender bias among survivors mentioned by name. Here, out of 1,247 survivors studied, 50 (4%) were women and the remaining 1,197 (96%) were men. Furthermore, among the women, only 10 were mentioned by name—which, when computed as a percentage of the total survivors population, yields a dismal .8%.

These statistics clearly establish gender bias against female mention and identification by name. Evidence from other areas of the obituary pages further substantiated this bias. Here I give an example from what is referred to in the Egyptian obituary pages as *shukr* (thanks)—a column or section of the obituary pages where families of the deceased publicly thank those who participated in the funeral or other mourning ceremonies. Mourning ceremonies are traditionally sex-segregated. Women visit with female members of the deceased family during a 3-day mourning period, usually at the family's residence. Men, on the other hand, attend the funeral procession, the religious ceremony (be it at a mosque or church[3]), the internment (usually restricted to very immediate male family members), and, in most cases, a one-evening

---

[3]Christian women would most likely be allowed to attend the religious ceremonies because, in general, they are not barred from attending church. The situation among the muslims is slightly different because women, again in general, do not participate in the public practice of religion (e.g., the Friday mosque prayers).

ceremony at the family residence. Men's mourning ceremonies are therefore all held in public,[4] whereas women's are held in the privacy of the home with other family members and friends by their side.

Among the few rare cases of deceased women mentioned by name in 1938 was the obituary of Miss Amina *hanim* Riad, part of which is given in Obituary 3.

> Obituary 3: Passed into God's mercy Miss Amina *hanim* Riad; **daughter** of the late Ali *bey* Riad; **maternal aunt** of *Amiralay* Ahmad Riad *bey*, former [retired] Inspector of Cairo Prison Administration, Ali *effendi* Riad, of the Notables, Mohammad *effendi* Fikri, retired Railway Station [official], *sheik* Mohammad Zaki Badr, teacher, Mohammad *effendi* Labib Hasanein, teacher; **maternal aunt** of the wife of Salih *effendi* Kamal and Abdel Aziz *effendi* Badr, teacher; **paternal aunt** of . . . [OB#38; 3/9/38][5]

Obviously the deceased was not married: she was given the title *anisa* "Miss," and no husband or offspring were mentioned. She was identified first as daughter of the late Ali *bey* Riad; next as the maternal aunt of a number of males and one female identified as the wife of Salih *effendi* Kamal (i.e., she is identified by the offsprings of her siblings). Although there was nothing especially unusual about this particular obituary, I quote it because 3 days later (3/12/1938), two *shukr* announcements appeared: one from her sisters, who incidentally were never directly mentioned in the obituary only indirectly through the mention of their offspring as just explained, and the other is from *Amiralay* Ahmad Riad (the first mentioned nephew) and the rest of the family. I quote for illustration a portion of each.

> Obituary 4: The sisters of the late[6] Amina *hanim* Riad offer their deep thanks to those who consoled them in the loss of their dear one, and they ask God to spare them any misfortune in relation to their dear ones.

---

[4]Even the one-evening mourning ceremony is often held outside the home. A tent of a sort is often built to allow male visitors and officials to pay their respects to the family of the deceased as represented by its male members.

[5]Comments on the translation: Inspector of the Cairo Prison Administration is a translation of *mufatish maslahat sugun misr*. In Arabic *misr* is ambiguous in that it is used to refer to Egypt and to Cairo. I opted to translate it as Cairo here, but it could very well be Egypt. One would have to check the records and see how the term was applied at the time and whether there were two separate administrations. I have also used the term *Notables* to translate *alaᶜyan*, a term also used to refer to a class very much similar to the notables in the West. Finally in Obituary 3, "Major General" is a translation for *liwaa'*.

[6]"The late" here translates *almaghfur laha* (lit.: the forgiven one).

> Obituary 5: *Amiralay* Ahmad Riad and the rest of the family thank all
> those who have consoled them in their misfortune, the passing away of
> their dear one,[7] and they especially mention their Excelencies: *Major
> General* [liwa'] Mohammad Haidar *pasha*, Director General of the Prison
> Administration, Mahmoud Sami *pasha*, Abdel Rahim Fahmi *pasha*, . . .

The first *shukr* came from the sisters of the deceased. Their names were
not mentioned but the deceased name was. The *shukr* was addressed to
women only, which was not reflected in the English translation but was
indicated in Arabic by the morpho-syntax of the announcement. All
verbal and pronominal inflections are marked for feminine plural—the
inflection used for exclusively female reference. The second shukr came
from the family, which appears to be headed by *Amiralay* Ahmad Riad,
who was obviously mentioned by name. It was addressed to all those
who participated in the mourning ceremonies but gave specific mention
by name to some of these participants: all were men, mostly with titles
(e.g., *pasha*) or in influential positions. But it did not mention the name of
the deceased. The morpho-syntax of Obituary 5 uses the masculine plural
instead—the inflection used in reference to all male groups as well as
groups inclusive of both sexes. Thus, the contrast between these two *shukr*
announcements provides further support for gender bias in favor of men
with respect to accessibility and identification in this public domain.[8]

But that was 1938, and we would expect a different picture to
emerge if we examine the population as a whole (i.e., all 6 years). Before
doing so, however, I briefly discuss two obituaries from 1988 in order to
illustrate some of the changes that took place in the representation of
women so as to present a more balanced picture of the situation.

> Obituary 6: Passed into God's Mercy *alustatha* <u>Kazim Beshir Hamid</u>,
> former Director of Rushdy Technical School; **wife** of *alustath* Ahmad
> Fahmi, former Director of Preparatory Education; **mother** of *alsayyida*
> <u>Shery</u> wife of *Mr.* Ahmad Mikkawi, Consultant at the Arab League;
> **daughter** of the late *ustath* Beshir Hamid, former Under-Secretary of
> Education; **sister** of *Dr.* Mustafa Beshir, a forensic doctor in Saudia,
> *alsayyida* <u>Safiyya Beshir</u> at the Mohammad Karim Schools wife of the
> late Mahmoud Elgohari; **in-law** of the late Mr. Sabir Hassan, Director of
> the Shabrawishi Factories; **niece** of . . . [#563; 4/5/88; 36 lines]

---

[7]The translation here reflects the Arabic *faqidatihim* "their lost one," which
sounds quite awkward in English.

[8]In accordance with the editorial policy adopted for this volume to mention
women before men, the sisters' *shukr* is mentioned and discussed before the
"family's" (i.e., male members). However, in the newspaper column, the
family's shukr appears first and the sisters' second (i.e., below it), which, I
believe, is significant in that it attributes more prominence to the family's (=
male members) *shukr*.

Obituary 7: Passed into the heavenly glories *engineer* Michel Iskandar Youssef, former General Director of The Arab Company for Cotton Ginning; **husband** of the late <u>Mary Halim</u> in Ab[n]oub; **father** of *Dr.* Nagi at the Suez Canal University [who is] husband of *alsayyida* <u>Jean Iskandar</u>, *Dr.* <u>Mona</u> at School Health in Talkha [who is] wife of *Dr.* Munir Michel, *Dr.* <u>Hoda</u> wife of Engineer Wadi^c Malti in America, *Dr.* <u>Amira</u> wife of *Dr.* Atef Halim in Libya, and *Dr.* <u>Dalal</u> wife of Dr. Mugib Girgis in Libya; **brother** of *Dr.* Fouad in Talkha, *engineer* Youssef, *sister* Munira, *producer* <u>Kiria</u>, <u>the wife of Saleh Mishrei</u>, George Naguib, and the late Khalil Nashed; **husband of the sister** of the late Fayez and the late Unsi, Nabil, a dealer in Tawfiqiya, Amir in Delta [Company] for Ginning, and *Dr.* Kamal in England, and their sisters. Funeral procession was held yesterday, and mourning ceremonies are held at home 247 Gumhouria St in Mansoura. [#566; 4/5/88; 23 lines]

The first is an obituary of a Muslim woman, the second a Christian man. They differ little in terms of how people are identified. In both, the deceased were identified by their full names (Kazim Beshir Hamid in Obituary 6 and Michel Iskandar Youssef in Obituary 7), their titles (*ustatha* in Obituary 6 and engineer in Obituary 7), their jobs (former director of the Rushdy Technical School in Obituary 6 and former director of the Arab Company for Cotton Ginning in Obituary 7). Their spouses are then mentioned with their own names. The husband in Obituary 6 was mentioned by title and occupation; the wife in Obituary 7 was not, most likely because she did not have one. This assumption can be further confirmed by looking at the survivors. Here many women were mentioned by occupation and by professional titles as well. (I underlined women's names for those not familiar with Arabic names.) In Obituary 6 spouses of survivors were mentioned. Husbands of female survivors were, as expected, mentioned very often. But wives of male survivors were now mentioned as well; and when they were, they were also identified by their titles and occupations.

Does this mean that equity had been achieved in 1988? Statistics from the survivors data, not as yet available, will hopefully answer this question. At this time, however, the examples in Obituaries 6 and 7 can at least illustrate where women's representation is heading and how the change will, most likely, proceed. But to answer the question of equity between the sexes, a look at the total population statistics is needed. However, I ignore the survivors population and report on my findings with respect to the deceased population only.

Table 2.1 shows that 84% of the deceased population were identified with their own (given) names, and a substantial 210 (16%) were mentioned without. But when broken down by sex, these statistics became much more impressive because 210 deceased persons not

Table 2.1. Name and Sex for Total Population.

Name	Female	Male	Total
No	210 (38.3%)	0 (0 %)	210 (15.7%)
Yes	338 (61.7%)	789 (100%)	1,127 (84.3%)
Totals	548 (100%)	789 (100%)	1,337 (100%)

mentioned by name were all women. Of the 548 females represented, 338 (61.7%) were mentioned with their own names and 210 (38.3%) without; thus almost 40% of the women had no names. Again, the figures became more impressive when compared with the men's, where of the 789 obituaries of men none were represented without names.

These figures then reduce all variation in the use of names to the identification of women because men were always identified by their own (first) names, and name avoidance becomes a strategy applicable only in the identification of women, thus confirming the gender basis of this variation.

To explain this discrepancy, I take the position that the representation of people in the obituaries is in some way a reflection of the way they are, and possibly wish to be, perceived in the society. In the case of the deceased, it is the way their families wish to have them be perceived, or think they would have liked to have been perceived by the public, specifically, by readers of the obituary pages who would naturally include family, friends, colleagues, acquaintances, among others.[9] The decisions are ultimately made by the families, within the context of the various social groups and communities in which both they and their deceased are (or have been) a part. These groups, then, become the audience to whom the obituaries are addressed.

If this is so, some major factors that may affect people's decisions in identifying their deceased include their religious affiliation, the geographical location from which they come, their socioeconomic status and that of their families, and possibly the age of the deceased. I argued elsewhere (Eid, 1994b) that religious affiliation, location, and status impose certain traditions and modes of behavior on their membership, which eventually become expected norms that serve to identify and symbolically represent that community. But symbols can be

---

[9]Of course this relates to the "who writes the obituaries?" question and the kinds of considerations involved in the obituary writing process—a question addressed in more detail in the longer version of this project.

both linguistic and nonlinguistic. Nonlinguistic symbols include dress, for example, which can easily identify people on the basis of these three variables. Linguistic symbols include not only speech patterns and styles characteristic of various regions, classes, and racial and ethnic groups but also forms of address, the use of names and titles, and other forms of identification. Name avoidance (or the identification of people without their names) can therefore be viewed as a linguistic symbol that serves to identify women, for it is only women whose identity, and hence their name, appears to be eclipsed and made dependent on someone else's (usually a man). In the next section, I look at the effect of the two variables (Time and Religion) on this variation.

GENDER INEQUALITY: TIME AND RELIGIOUS AFFILIATION

To assess the effect of time, the data are broken down by year. Table 2.2 provides figures on women mentioned with and without a name obtained from each year separately. They show a steady increase in the number of deceased women identified by their own names. The percentage of women represented by their names has more than doubled during this period, starting with 37.5% in 1938 and ending with 87.4% in 1988.

Table 2.3 reports the increase per decade, again measured in percentage point difference. The largest increase (17.2%) occurred in the period from 1968-1978. This decade can, therefore, be said to constitute a turning point in the history of female representation; it was the period with the highest increase in the percentage of families representing their deceased by name. This result confirms my initial hypothesis, and can be explained historically on the basis of the socioeconomic and cultural changes that took place in post-1952 Egypt—changes in the status of women triggered by government policies on education, employment, family and health care, among other things. The following quotes from Hooglund (1991) describe some changes that could have impacted the status of women, hence their image and public identity.

> The proportion of the population with some secondary education more than doubled between 1960 and 1976; the number of people with some university education nearly tripled. . . . Women made great educational gains: the percentage of women with preuniversity education grew more than 300% while women with University education grew more than 600%.

Table 2.2. Female Identification by Name Per Year.

Name	1938	1948	1958	1968	1978	1988
Yes	21 (37.5%)	51 (46.8%)	52 (54.2%)	60 (60.0%)	71 (77.2%)	83 (87.4%)
No	35 (62.5%)	58 (53.2%)	44 (45.8%)	40 (40.0%)	21 (22.8%)	12 (12.6%)
Total	56	109	96	100	92	95

Table 2.3. Increase in Women's Representation by Name.

1938-1948	1948-1958	1958-1968	1968-1978	1978-1988
9.3%	7.4%	5.8%	17.2%	10.2%

In the first ten years following the 1952 Revolution, spending on higher
education increased 400%. Between academic years 1951-52 and 1978-
79, student enrollment in public universities grew nearly 1400%. . . .
The total number of female college students had doubled; by 1985-86
women accounted for 32% of all students. (p. 147)

The change in the obituaries during the 1968 to 1978 period can,
therefore, be viewed as a result of changes that took place in post-1952
Egypt.

Religion, the second variable examined, turned out to be one of
the strongest predictors of identification by name. Table 2.4 gives a
breakdown of the deceased population by Religion and Name, first in
relation to the total population then in relation to the female population.
Christians are less likely to represent their deceased without a name—
only 9% of them did, as compared to 20% among the Muslims. The
Muslim population shows more deceased women mentioned without
than with their names (53% to 47%), thus accounting for the high
percentage of women identified without their names.

Examination of the effect of this variable on women's
identification over time reveals an even more interesting picture. Table
2.5 shows that the trend in both Christian and Muslim populations is
towards an increased identification of women by name. But they also
show the distance between the two populations. The Christian
population started with a 65% female representation by name in 1938
and grew to a 95% in 1988, whereas the Muslim population started with
an initial 20% and ended with an 81.5% representation by name in 1988,
significantly below the Christian population.

Figure 2.1 provides a graphic view of the percentages of women
identified by name for each year. It shows a steady increase in the
female population toward representation by name. But it also shows
varying degrees of distance between the two religious groups as well as
the trajectories of change.

Table 2.4. Name of Deceased in Relation to Religion.

Name	Total Population		Female Population	
	Muslim	Christian	Muslim	Christian
No	164 (20%)	46 (8.9%)	164 (52.9%)	46 (19.4%)
Yes	656 (80%)	469 (91.1%)	146 (47.1%)	191 (80.6%)
Total	820 (61.3%)	515 (38.5%)	310 (100%)	237 (100%)

Table 2.5. Religion and Women Identified by Name.

Religion	1938	1948	1958	1968	1978	1988
Christian	13 (65%)	31 (67.4%)	43 (86%)	30 (81.1%)	35 81.4%)	39 (95.1%)
Muslim	7 (20%)	20 (31.8%)	9 (19.6%)	30 (47.7%)	36 (73.5%)	44 (81.5%)

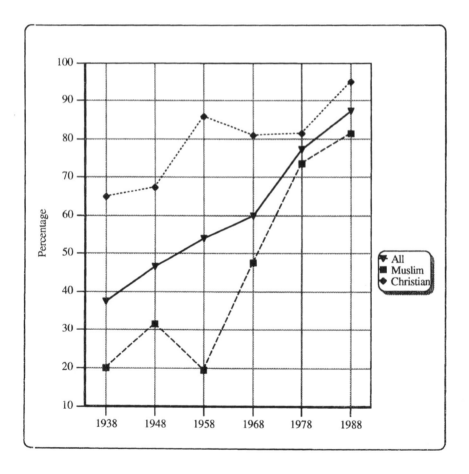

Figure 2.1. Women identified by name:
Religious affiliation and time effects

VARIATION IN TITLES

The previous discussion establishes the gender basis of name avoidance as a strategy for identifying people in the obituaries, and the effect of religious affiliation (another form of identification) on this variation. And although name avoidance, strongest in 1938, decreased over time, it was still not totally abandoned by 1988. Public identity as evidenced by the obituaries can be said to depend on one's sex and religion, among other things.

The question of public identity is communicated in the obituaries through two other linguistic variables: titles and occupation. Table 2.6 provides a summary of the title and occupation data for the population broken down by Sex.

Titles are divided into two types: professional and social. Professional titles need no explanation; they are basically derived from one's profession: doctor, professor, general, engineer, and so on. In view of the overlap between an occupation name and a title derived from that occupation, I followed the following procedure in coding title versus occupation. Because titles in Arabic precede the name, a profession is counted as title if it occupies that position; it is counted as an occupation if it occurs after the name. Social titles refer to some aspect of social status or identity; they can be personal or marital (*sayid* "Mr.," *anisa* "Miss," *Haram* "Mrs.," *armala* "widower, fem."), religious (*sheikh, muqaddis, Hagg*), honorific (*pasha, bey, effendi*), and son on.

The majority of women and men, as Table 2.6 shows, are identified by a title: 53% of the women and 62% of the men, which points to the cultural significance of titles in Egyptian/Arab society in general. But the difference between the sexes becomes apparent when examining the type of title used with each. Table 2.6 shows 30% of the men are identified with a professional title, but less than 2% of the women have a professional title. And although social titles are used extensively with both sexes, they are more important for women than for men. Almost all the women identified with a title are identified with a social title, specifically 98% of them as compared to only 72% of the men.

A comparison of the data from professional titles and occupation provides an insight into the relative importance of the two in the identification of people in the obituaries. Of the men, 54% are identified with an occupation, but only 30% have a professional title (see Table 2.6). For women, the situation is dismal on both counts: Only 4% are identified with an occupation and less than 2% with professional titles. For both sexes, however, the number of deceased identified by occupation is higher than the number identified by professional titles. This points to the importance of occupation in establishing public identity. If this is so, then

Table 2.6. Titles and Occupation in Relation to Sex.

	Title		Professional Title		Social Title		Occupation	
	Female	Male	Female	Male	Female	Male	Female	Male
Yes	317	527	5	158	312	380	23	428
	(53%)	(62%)	(2%)	(30%)	(98%)	(72%)	(4%)	(54%)
No	231	262	312	369	5	145	425	361
	(47%)	(38%)	(98%)	(70%)	(2%)	(28%)	(96%)	(46%)
Total	548	789	317	527	317	525	548	789

occupation becomes the way to public identity, and we would expect the number of women identified by their occupation to increase over time. We would also expect women to be identified by occupation prior to their being identified by professional titles.

Tables 2.7 and 2.8 provide the necessary support here. Professional titles for deceased women appear only in 1988, where 5 out of 52 women identified by a title had a professional rather than social title. Prior to that point, none of the women had professional titles. Table 2.8 shows the earliest instance of a woman identified by an occupation appeared quite a bit earlier in 1948. The number continued to increase but remained quite small on the whole.

The picture that emerges from the results obtained so far supports the idea that public identity may very well be tied to occupation. For women, this may be the only route to a public and independent identity. Such a conclusion would have to await a more detailed analysis of the title and occupation data.

CONCLUSION

So far in this research I have established that uses of the linguistic variables studied (names, titles, occupations) depend on sex, but other factors (such as religious affiliation) also have a strong effect on this variation, at least in the case of name avoidance. These same factors are also hypothesized to have a strong impact on women's public identity. I hope continued research in this area would allow us to determine the overall effect of these variables on women's public identity and to explain why they affect it the way they do.

Table 2.7. Professional Titles by Year and Sex.

	1938		1948		1958		1968		1978		1988	
	Female	Male	Female	Male	Female	Male	Female	Male	Female	Male	Female	Male
Yes	0	6 (8%)	0	11 (11%)	0	26 (31%)	0	34 (39%)	0	41 (45%)	5 (10%)	40 (48%)
No	30	73 (92%)	67	91 (89%)	58	58 (69%)	56	54 (61%)	54	50 (55%)	47 (90%)	43 (52%)
Total	30	79	67	102	58	84	56	88	54	91	52	83

Table 2.8. Occupation by Year and Sex.

	1938		1948		1958		1968		1978		1988	
	Female	Male	Female	Male	Female	Male	Female	Male	Female	Male	Female	Male
Yes	0	52	1 (1%)	63 (48%)	2 (2%)	64 (45%)	7 (7%)	84 (62%)	5 (5%)	77 (53%)	8 (8%)	88 (61%)
No	56	40 (43%)	108 (99%)	67 (52%)	94 (98%)	77 (55%)	93 (93%)	52 (38%)	87 (95%)	69 (47%)	87 (92%)	56 (39%)
Total	56	92	109	130	96	141	100	136	92	146	95	144

REFERENCES

Adler, M. K. (1978). *Naming and addressing: A sociolinguistic study*. Hamburg: Buske.

Eid, M. (1994a). Hidden women: Gender inequality in 1938 Egyptian obituaries. In R. Rammuny & D. Parkinson (Eds.), *Investigating Arabic: Linguistic, pedagogical, and literary studies in honor of Ernest N. McCarus* (pp. 111-136). Columbus, OH: Greyden Press.

Eid, M. (1994b). "What's in a name?" Women in Egyptian obituaries. In Y. Suleiman (Ed.), *Arabic sociolinguistics: Issues and perspectives* (pp. 81-100). London: Curzon Press.

Hooglund, E. (1991). The society and its environment. In H. C. Metz (Ed), *Egypt: A country study* (pp. 91-153). Washington, DC: Library of Congress Federal Research Division.

Smith, P. M. (1985). *Language, the sexes and society*. New York: Basil Blackwell.

3

THE POWER OF WOMEN'S VOICES IN THE PRACTICE OF *CHISMEANDO*

JOAN KELLY HALL

> True life is not lived where great external changes take place—where
> people move about, clash, fight and slay one another—it is lived only
> where these tiny, tiny infinitesimally small changes occur
>   —Leo Tolstoy

Everyday face-to-face interactive practices appear to be, perhaps because of their ubiquity, rather ordinary and uneventful. Studies however, of such practices (e.g., Goodwin, 1992; Hall, 1993b), have shown them to be constitutive of a mutually shaping, locally situated struggle between the sociocultural forces embedded in their linguistic and paralinguistic elements and the individual participants. There has also been a focused interest in the examination of the power embedded in the control or manipulation of the linguistic and paralinguistic elements of oral practices (see e.g., Goodwin, 1992; Hall 1993b) as well as a parallel interest in looking at how larger sociopolitical and sociohistorical processes are constituted in everyday talk.

In what follows, I briefly summarize the notion of interactive practice as it is used here and the research on the nature of gossiping as a social practice. This is followed by a short description of the practice and the group of women participants. I then examine the sociocultural knowledge embedded in the stories told and the uses of two intonation patterns in the storytelling. Finally, I discuss these moments and the practice itself both in terms of its importance to this group of women and of the larger issues of sociopolitics and situated action, and suggest areas for further study.

The study reported here is part of these larger research interests. My primary intent is to show that the practice of *chismeando*[1] as defined and engaged in by a group of women from the Dominican Republic is an important sociocultural and sociopolitical activity. I argue that in this practice, the women collectively remember and create sociocultural knowledge important to living their daily lives. I examine in particular, the ways in which these women use two different intonation patterns to foreground and create *chisme* (gossip). I argue that the uses of the formulae, which on one level may seem inconsequential, are important sociopolitical acts by which the women actively constitute or maintain the social rules by which they live their lives. My empirical data challenge any claim to a universal meaning of these paralinguistic conventions, demonstrating instead that meanings of these (and other interactive) patterns emerge from the dialogue between the larger sociohistorical forces embedded in the practice and their contextually situated uses by particular groups of people and individuals in those groups (Bakhtin, 1986; Morson & Emerson, 1990).

THE NATURE OF INTERACTIVE PRACTICES

Conversation, telling stories, telling jokes, gossiping, and other similar behaviors are known as *interactive practices*. Interactive practices are goal-directed, recurring episodes of face-to-face interaction that are significant to the establishment and maintenance of our social groups and communities. Participation in these practices is mediated by particular symbolic tools and other communicative resources (e.g., language, intonation patterns, gestures, body stance, voice qualities, etc.) that provide structuring frameworks for the creation, articulation, and management of collective social histories (Vygotsky, 1978; Wertsch,

---

[1]Although the substantive *chismear* may seem a more grammatically correct choice, I chose to use the word *chismeando* to frame what the women are doing as it is the word they used in describing what they were doing.

1991). These resources include lexical and syntactic choices, participation structures, act sequences, and prosodic and other formulae to signal opening, transitional, and closing moves. Communicating meaning in an interactive practice depends on our shared understanding of the conventional (i.e., historical) ways in which the resources get used. It is this conventionality that to some degree binds us to particular ways of using the resources in our practices. Their actual meaning, however, emerges from the ways in which we use them at a particular moment. Bakhtin's (1986; Morson & Emerson, 1990) notion of dialogicality captures the tension that exists at any moment in a practice between the sociohistorical, conventionalized nature of the communicative resources, and their locally situated, emergent uses during the practice itself. It is the simultaneous attention to these resources and their locally-situated uses that can reveal the myriad ways groups formulate voices in relation to larger social forces (Gal, 1989).

GOSSIPING AS A SOCIAL PRACTICE

The study of "gossiping" has generated a great deal of scholarly interest in a variety of disciplines (e.g., Brenneis, 1984; Coates, 1989; Connerton, 1989; Eckert, 1990; Eder & Enke, 1991; Gluckman, 1963; Goodwin, 1992; Hall, 1993a, 1993b; Hannerz, 1967; Haviland, 1977). In these studies, the content of gossip is defined as a certain kind of talk about a socially unacceptable act that happened to or was instigated by a person not present at the time of the talk or is acted toward as if she were absent (i.e., she is talked about in the third person). Its primary function is to serve as a forum for the display of social control within which group members, by talking about others, are able to exert collective power over each other and keep each other's social behavior in check. Through posing and responding to real social dilemmas in this practice, people develop, display, and sustain their sociocultural competence.

The study presented here confirms earlier conclusions, and extends the analysis by demonstrating the kind of information that is contained in the stories and its social significance to these women, and the situated, dynamic nature of these processes (i.e., how the [re]creation of significant sociocultural knowledge is interactionally realized).

CHISMEANDO

Sociocultural Context and Participants

The data that form the basis of this study are part of a larger audiotaped data set I collected in the town of San Cristóbal, Dominican Republic during a 3-month stay in 1989. The Dominican Republic is a Spanish-speaking country, and shares the island of Hispaniola in the Caribbean with the country of Haiti. San Cristóbal is the capital of the province of the same name and lies about 28 kilometers to the southwest of Santo Domingo, the capital of the country.

The data consist of 55 minutes of audiotaped interaction. The woman with whom I lived, who is also member of the women's barrio and who lived closer to the center of town, assisted me in the transcription and analysis. The women themselves also helped me. The women and a number of townspeople also participated in some semi-structured interviews conducted during the 3-month period in 1989 and in a follow-up visit in 1990. These are included as secondary data sources.

The country is poor and about 75% of its population are the lower middle and working classes. Most of the people are mulatto; 25% are White or hispanic (15%), and Black (10%) (Wiarda & Kryzanek, 1992). The participants in this study as well as the majority of the population of the town of San Cristóbal are mulatto and members of the lower middle and working classes at the time of the study.

The women ranged in age from about 13 to 22. At the time of the study, most attended school, either during the day or at night, and a few had jobs as house or laundry maids in middle- and upper middle-class homes located closer to the center of town. A few studied English at one of the several English-language institutes located around town. Most hoped to marry and remain in San Cristóbal, although a few had aspirations to go to the United States to live and work. Only one, the oldest, was married. She had two children and was married to the brother of one of the other participants.

I lived among and interacted with the women for about 2 months, joining in some of the *chismeando* sessions, and building a level of confianza (trust) before I asked to record them. They made me feel like a friend and confidante. I am not unaware that my status as an American may have colored our interactions in ways not visible to me.

According to the women, two criteria guided a decision as to whom one could engage in *chismeando:* those with whom one had *confianza* and those whose social power was perceived to be more or less equal. Relevant components of the women's establishment and maintenance of *confianza* included similarity and proximity of living conditions and a shared understanding of the social rules against which the reported displays of improper behavior were evaluated. The women all lived in the same barrio and considered themselves good friends among whom existed a high level of *confianza*. Age and gender did not seem to be a strong factor in deciding with whom one could share *confianza*. Although the practice reported on here was engaged in entirely by women, no one considered *chismeando* to be solely a woman's activity.

Sociocultural Knowledge Constructed in *Chismeando*

Presented here is an overview of the sociocultural knowledge embedded in the *chismeando* stories told by the women. Such an examination provides a window into the sociocultural knowledge these women considered important to the living of their daily lives as members of their community.

All talk considered by the women to be *chisme* concerned some questionable social behavior of another person who was either not present during the interaction, acted towards as if she or he were not present, or of people passing by the group while they were engaged in *chismeando*. The behavior talked about did not have to actually occur; rather, it at least had to be a possible occurrence.

The formation and maintenance of interpersonal relationships both with each other and with men were the primary focus of the stories. Three behaviors most frequently gossiped about were women being with men in particular places where and/or when they shouldn't be, women wearing borrowed items such as shoes and items of clothing around town and damaging them, and women acting "stuck up" (i.e., seeming to be unwilling to talk with the other members of the community). Other less frequent topics included unmarried women who had gotten pregnant, couples who had gotten into fights, and boyfriends who flirted with other women.

In all stories told, the women were always referred to by name and all were members of the barrio where the gossipers lived. Most frequently mentioned were women members of their group. Interestingly, when men featured as characters in the stories, they remained anonymous, being referred to as un *muchacho* (a boy) or *el/ese novio* (the/that boyfriend). Naming of specific men in *chismeando* was not necessary to the telling or creating of scandal. Instead, it was the naming of women and the suggestion of some kind of association with a (any) man either at a time that was inappropriate or in a place that was considered improper and thus worthy of being talked about.

Two kinds of places served as settings in these stories: those suggested to be improper because of the time of the meeting, at night, and those considered to be improper because of the kind of place it was. Some of the specific places mentioned in the stories in which women were said to have been seen with *un muchacho* at night and thus used to suggest socially improper behavior included "down by the river," "on the corner by Ramoncito's," and "at the beach." The women stated that these places, by themselves, were not considered inappropriate places for women to be. Rather, it was women being in them, or suggested to be in them, with men at inappropriate times that was considered scandalous.

Two places were frequently cited and when mentioned generated heightened audience reaction. One was the town of Hatillo, a small town about 12 kilometers outside of San Cristóbal, and the site of field headquarters for a number of government engineering projects. This distinction brought to the town an increased population of construction workers of national and international origin, and as such, Hatillo had a reputation in the town as a place with wild and corrupt ways. Another place important in the making of scandal and often used as a setting of stories was the Bar Dorado located in the center of San Cristóbal.

Example 1 shows the use of the place to suggest a display of improper behavior by one of the members of the group. According to this story, Susana, a girl about whom much *chisme* occurred, was said to have been seen sitting in Dorado, a place considered to be filled with *tigres* (tigers—men of ill-repute) and loose women. It was certainly not a place for a proper Dominican woman to be. By suggesting that Susana was seen there, the teller of the story implies that Susana was engaged in some kind of scandalous behavior. The frequency with which these places were mentioned in chismeando and the heightened responses their naming called forth clearly indicate their social importance in the lives of these women.

Example 1[2]
```
1. Mari:   bueno Lola a mi no me gusta el chisme pero tú no sabes que
2.         Susana anoche andaba por ahí, muchacha, y esa muchacha
3.         estaba=
```

---

[2]Pseudonyms are used for all participants, both as tellers of the stories and characters within them. Transcription conventions include: ⌈⌊ to indicate overlapping talk; : to indicate vowel elongation; = to indicate connected talk (i.e., no pause between the utterances); ( ) to indicate incomprehensible talk; ↑ and ↓ to indicate rising and falling intonation, respectively. The English translation follows each example.

4. Lola: =quién=
5. Mari: =o Susana=
6. Lola: =↑có:: ⌈ ↓ mo
7. Otra: ⌊ Su⌈ sa::na
8. Mari: ⌊ (digo yo) Justina y Susana estaban en la
9.   iglesia y fui a la iglesia en la iglesia qué yo la estaba
10.   buscando para que fuéramos a la heladería y cuando yo
11.   pasé por Dorado estaba Susana sentada en ↑Do:ra::↓do=
12. Lola: =↑o::: ⌈↓o::
13. Otras: ⌈⌊↑a:::↓y::
14.   ⌊↑có:::↓mo::=
15. Arlene: =para que ↑tú↓ve:↓a para que ↑tú ve:↓a

1. Mari: well Lola I don't like gossip but don't you know that
2.   Susana last night was walking around, girl, and that girl
3.   was=
4. Lola: =who=
5. Mari: =oh Susana=
6. Lola: =↑wha::⌈↓:t
7. Other: ⌊Su ⌈↑sa::na
8. Mari: ⌊(I say) Justina and Susana were at
9.   church and I went to the church in the church what I was
10.   looking for her so we could go to the ice cream shop and
            when I
11.   passed by Dorado there was Susana sitting in ↑Do:ra::↓do=
12. Lola: =↑o::: ⌈↓o::
13. Others: ⌈ ⌊↑o:::↓::h
14.   ⌊↑wha:::↓::t=
15. Arlene: =so that ↑you'd see:↓her so that ↑you'd see:↓her

Coger prestado (borrowing items) was an important and frequently engaged in social activity by all members of the town and as such was an activity about which there was much potential for socially inappropriate behavior, making it a frequent topic in *chismeando*. Example 2 is about one such incident. In this story, as in many others, *coger prestado* is treated as an important and serious social activity, as it was one way the women worked creatively with their low economic resources to wear clothing items and accessories considered to be luxuries. Each invested in a few items, which they then treated as community resources by lending the items to each other. Thus, taking good care of items borrowed and appropriately responding to improper treatment given to one's belongings were important social rules used by the women in the evaluation of their own and others' behaviors.

In the following story, the fact that a woman had damaged a borrowed dress and still wore it "modeling" around town is offered and responded to as a socially inappropriate act.

Example 2
1. Arlene: ay pero ven acá ustedes no saben la última=
2. Mari: =cúal es la última
3. Arlene: viene Aidé ayer=
4. Lola: =Aidé ayer aquí la de allí ⌈de la esquina
5. Arlene: ⌊modela↑:: ⌈ndo
6. Mari::   ⌊la ↑hija ne↓gra=
7. Arlene: =sí sí con el vestido azul que yo le presté ↑modelan↓do
8. Morena: y te lo rompió
9. Arlene: y yo me quedé callada

1. Arlene: oh but come here you don't know the latest=
2. Mari: =what's the latest
3. Arlene: Aidé comes yesterday=
4. Lola: Aidé yesterday here the one from over there from the corner
5. Arlene: ⌊model↑:: ing
6. Mari:
                                                ⌈   ⌊↑the
           Black gi↓rl=   ⌈
7. Arlene: =yeah yeah with the blue dress that I lent her ↑ model↓ing
8. Morena: and she tore it on you
9. Arlene: and I kept quiet

The *chismeando* stories reveal much about what was valued in a man. That men quite often had multiple concurrent relationships with women seemed an accepted fact; more salient behaviors in evaluating social appropriateness was whether men supported their families in some way and did not inflict physical violence on the women or children. Example 3 shows how the possibility of socially improper behavior by one man was brought forth for discussion and evaluated by the women as he passed by their group. The fact that he brought home some of his wages to his mother and siblings was evaluated quite positively by the group and used to dissuade others from providing *chisme* about him. Mari, in fact, tells the others twice to "shut up" since he is "the best boy."

Example 3
1. Mari: ay espérate ahí viene Ram wages to his mother and
2. Lola: es muy chévere ese muchacho el mejor muchacho es Ramón
3. Mari: =cállense que ahí viene Ramón el mejor muchacho
4.   es Ramón es un muchacho muy serio cállense
5.   que ahí viene Ramón ⌈el mejor muchacho
6. Lola: ⌊cuando cobra lleva cuarto a su casa
7.   le da cuarto a su mamá y a sus hermanos=
8. Mari: =él es muy bueno

1. Mari: oh wait, here comes Ramón fighting for Arlene
2. Lola: he's great that boy the best boy is Ramón
3. Mari: =shut up 'cause here comes Ramón the best boy
4.   is Ramón he is a very serious boy shut up
5.   'cause here comes Ramón ⌈the best boy
6. Lola: ⌊when he gets money he brings
       some to his house
7.   he give some to his mother and to his siblings=
8. Mari: =he is very good

Another important aspect of the social lives of these women as displayed and created in the practice of *chismeando* is religion. Religion often served as a criterion for deciding whether someone could be the subject of *chisme* and whether the inappropriate behavior said to be displayed by someone was actually possible. In Example 4, Mari uses the concept of religion to allay Lola's fears that she might figure as a protagonist in one of the *chismeando* stories. Mari uses the fact that Lola went to church to explain why the others would not consider her as a potential story character.

Example 4
1. Mari: ay Lola no hablando de ti que tú eres muy seria
2.   que tú vas a la iglesia no de ti no se puede hablar

1. Mari: oh Lola not speaking about you 'cause you are very serious
2.   'cause you go to church no you can't be talked about

In summary, the stories of *chismeando* are concerned with far more than idle chatter. They reveal the people, places, activities, and norms that frame the interpersonal relationships that are significant to the women of San Cristobal as they go about the business of living their everyday lives.

(Re)Creating *Chisme*

Important in the practice of *chismeando* is the varied use of two
intonation patterns, the phrase-final fall and the phrase-final rise,[3] to
bring forth the most significant part of the *chisme* story, the alleged
improprietous act. The two are not determined by what follows their
uses, as the responses to both types of utterances were the same,
exclamations of incredulity, and so on. Rather, it is the type of text,
related versus *created chisme*, by which the distinction is made. In other
words, when the socially inappropriate act is clearly expressed in the
lexicogrammatical content of the utterance, the intonation falls at the
end. At these moments, it seems to be taken for granted by the
storyteller that the impropriety is clearly expressed in what was said,
and the falling intonation alerts the others to attend to the propositional
content of the statement. Example 5 contains examples of these
utterances.

Example 5
1.   tiene como ↑cinco no::↓vios
2.   estaba Susana sentada en ↑Do:ra::↓do
3.   esta mañana ( ) a mi y a Arlene dizque que que ella va para
       ↑Ha:ti::↓llo

1.   she has like ↑five bo::y↓friends
2.   there was Susana sitting in ↑Do:ra::↓do
3.   this morning ( ) to me and Arlene it's said that that she's going to
       Ha:ti::↓llo

      The claim that a girl has five boyfriends, as in Line 1 of Example
5, for instance, seemed to be a taken-for-granted impropriety in the lives
of these women, and was intonationally expressed as a phrase-final fall.
That is, the falling intonation alerted the listeners to attend to the
propositional content of the utterance as it made explicit the social
behavior that was being judged. Line 2 is taken from Example 1 (Line
11) and occurred as the climax of the story told by Mari about Susana.
As mentioned earlier, that the Bar Dorado and the town Hatillo are
places of ill repute was common knowledge to the townspeople of San
Cristóbal and the mere mention of their names as sites of particular
behaviors made explicit the impropriety of the act committed (i.e., being

---

[3]These patterns are similar to what Bolinger (1989) called, respectively, Profile A,
whole distinguishing feature is an abrupt fall from the highlighted syllable, and
Profile B in which there is first a jump up to the accented syllable and then a
continuous gradual rise.

in these places). This pattern, the phrase-final fall, was used to *present chisme* (i.e., to bring forth and open for discussion, statements about improper displays of social behavior by certain community members). The impropriety was commonly known and agreed on among the women and contained in the propositional content of the utterance.

In the second intonation pattern used to present a claim of inappropriately displayed behavior, the utterances ended on the rise. In these utterances fewer, or no, details about the alleged behavior were given. Instead, the phrase-final rise of the utterance implied an improper display of some behavior that if performed by someone else or in some other place or time might not have been considered improper. Four examples of utterances ending on the rise are included in Example 6. In each of these utterances what was said does not indicate a particularly improper behavior and what preceded and followed each of these does not clarify the impropriety. The fact, for example, that Madelín was seen on a street corner with a boy was not, in itself, improper behavior. However, by ending the utterance on the rise the storyteller created the possibility of impropriety and intended for the other participants to interpret it as such, which in all cases they did, by responding with exclamations of surprise (*ay*) or incredulity (*cómo*). The use of rising intonation invited suspicion of scandalous behavior (i.e., what was said was to be interpreted as improperly displayed social behavior by the character in question). By using this pattern the women *created chisme* from otherwise unremarkable displays of social activity.

Example 6
1. yo ví a Madelín anoche en la esquina ahí donde Ramoncito con un mu↑cha::cho
2. que dejó el novio por ↑aquí::
3. tenía un panta↑ló::n
4. que era en la parcela que estaba a las horas de la noche con un mu↑cha:cho

1. I saw Madelín last night on the corner by Ramoncito's with a ↑bo::y
2. that she left her boyfriend ↑he::re
3. she had on a pair of ↑pa::nts
4. it was in the field that she was at night with a ↑bo:y

I suggest here that the women's knowledge and use of these two patterns constitute two strategies of sociopolitical economy (Gal, 1989). The first pattern, the phrase-final fall, used by a storyteller, signaled to the other women that what was contained in the propositional content of the utterance was to be interpreted as explicit display of improper behavior. By bringing forth and evaluating stories about others' behaviors in this way the women foregrounded important social issues, set themselves apart from these issues, and were thus able to reflect on and deal with the social conditions by which they lived their lives. Using this particular pattern in the telling of chisme stories the women, either as storyteller or respondent to the stories, *displayed* the sociocultural knowledge necessary to maintain their status as *bona fide* members of the group. At the same time, it made visible their individual stances toward the larger social world in which they lived (i.e., made visible the issues important to them in shaping theirs and the others' social lives).

The knowledge and use of the second intonation pattern, the phrase-final rise, is a significant interactive strategy that is potentially more powerful than the first in that by ending utterances on the rise the women were able to *create chisme* from social moments that could otherwise be viewed as harmless. Through the use of this pattern the women actively engendered skepticism about a particular person's social behavior, and thus had the potential to transform any social act into an impropriety and any community member into a perpetrator of scandalous behavior. One would not have had to break a social rule to be made a story character in *chismeando* as any social act or person could be made to seem improper just by virtue of the rising intonation.

The use of the rising intonational pattern in creating *chisme* is a powerful strategy available to these women for changing the course of theirs and others' lives. On the one hand, this power to transform someone into a perpetrator of impropriety by naming her as a character in unspecified displays of impropriety sets up a frame of expectations that facilitates the making of other, similar interpretations, and as a consequence, casts a web of suspicion about the person's status as a socially proper community member. On the other hand, knowing how to *create chisme* about someone else in this way can be used to shield one from being made a character by others. That is, the more competent one is at controlling and manipulating the creation of *chisme* about others, the more socially powerful she is likely to be. Thus, it is less likely that others will attempt to use that knowledge against her. Further study is, of course, needed to substantiate this claim, although see Hall (1993b), for a study that examines an individual's control and manipulation of some of the conventions of chismeando in such a way as to positively affect her status in the group.

One more point needs to be made about the importance of the two patterns of interest here: Their roles as powerful tools in the (re)construction of the social lives of these women in *chismeando* challenge any claim to some universal meaning residing in the patterns themselves. They challenge in particular the claims made by Lakoff

(1975) and Bolinger (1989), for example, that the use of the rising intonation pattern is a universal index of uncertainty, hesitation, tentativeness and indecisiveness, its use marking some psychological weakness in the user. This is clearly not the case here. As demonstrated, the use of the rising intonation is a strategy that does not reflect a level of self-doubt residing in the user about what is being said but actively and forcefully *engenders* uncertainty, or even more seriously, skepticism in the minds of the other women about the degree and kind of social propriety residing in the behaviors of particular community members. Those using this strategy in creating *chisme* reflect no hesitation or tentativeness in doing this. Rather, as I argued earlier, its use creates a level of social power in the hands of the user that can serve to help maintain or modify both her status and that of the person being presented as a character in a *chisme* story. At the very least, the women's uses of these two patterns reveal the significance of context in the interpretation and construction of meaning of these and other linguistic and paralinguistic resources used in interactive practices.

CONCLUSIONS

The practice of *chismeando* is important in the lives of the women studied. The stories told contain significant sociocultural information. Moreover, the ways the storytellers use two prosodic conventions in evaluating the social behavior of others allow them to display and create important sociocultural knowledge.

This study is significant in a number of ways. First, it provides an understanding of the important role that the practice of *chismeando* can play in the building of intragroup support as women make visible what they, collectively, consider to be important sociocultural knowledge. By participating in the display and creation of such knowledge, the women solidify their allegiance to each other as social group members. In addition to its intragroup importance, the practice of *chismeando* can play an important role for those who are not members of the group but aspire to be. Because there is significant sociocultural knowledge embedded within the stories—knowledge that is for the most part difficult to locate elsewhere—by engaging as audience to the practice, outgroup members can develop some of the sociocultural competence needed to become a legitimate member of the group or at the very least come to understand what it means to be a legitimate member of the group.

Moreover, the study shows that a degree of sociopolitical power is embedded in the competent uses of two seemingly insignificant paralinguistic conventions. Hymes (1974) pointed out that "the more a way of speaking has become shared and meaningful within a group, the more likely that crucial cues will be efficient, i.e., slight in scale" (p. 54). Such is the case examined here. Although these cues used by the women may seem unremarkable, the potential for power embedded in their use clearly makes competent engagement in the practice of *chismeando* of some political importance to the successful accomplishment of their everyday lives. That is, knowing how to both display and create social rules and knowledge are skills useful to the evaluation of one's own and others behavior in ways that help to maintain the social group and one's status within it.

The study also demonstrates how the meanings of two particular intonation patterns, the phrase-final rise and the phrase-final fall, are tied to their uses in locally situated sociocultural activities, calling into question any universal claims to their meanings. It thus provides empirical support for Eckert and McConnell-Ginet's (1992) statement that such strategies can only be interpreted and evaluated in the contexts of their uses. It also provides evidence of an important sociopolitical activity in which powerful linguistic behaviors are used by women. The women's speech makes problematic the perspective that gossiping is mere solidarity-building "idle talk" (Holmes, 1993). The evidence presented here suggests otherwise and points to the need for a more situated, contextual study of language use in which such dimensions as the relationships among the participants, their social identities and roles played, and the social goal(s) brought to and negotiated in the interaction are taken into account.

REFERENCES

Bakhtin, M. M. (1986). *Speech genres and other late essays* (C. Emerson & M. Holquist, Eds.; V. W. McGee, Trans.). Austin: University of Texas Press.

Bolinger, D. (1989). *Intonation and its uses*. Stanford, CA: Stanford University Press.

Brenneis, D. (1984). Grog and gossip in Bhatgaon: Style and substance in Fiji Indian conversation. *American Ethnologist, 11,* 487-506.

Coates, J. (1989). Gossip revisited: Language in all-female groups. In J. Coates & D. Cameron (Eds.), *Women in their speech communities: New perspectives on language and sex* (pp 94-122). London: Longman.

Connerton, P. (1989). *How societies remember*. Cambridge: Cambridge University Press.

Eckert, P. (1990). Cooperative competition in adolescent "girl talk" *Discourse Processes, 11,* 91-122.

Eckert, P., & McConnell-Ginet, S. (1992). Think practically and look locally: Language and gender as community-based practice. *Annual Review of Anthropology, 21*, 461-490.

Eder, D., & Enke, J. (1991). The structure of gossip: Opportunities and constraints on collective expression among adolescents. *American Sociological Review, 56*, 494-508.

Gal, S. (1989). Language and political economy. *Annual Review of Anthropology, 18*, 345-367.

Gluckman, M. (1963). Gossip and scandal. *Current Anthropology, 4*, 307-315.

Goodwin, M. H. (1992). Orchestrating participation in events: Powerful talk Among African American girls. In K. Hall, M. Bucholtz, & B. Moonwoman (Eds.), *Locating power* (Vol. 1, pp. 182-196). Berkeley, CA: Berkeley's Women and Language Group.

Hall, J. K. (1993a). 'Tengo una bomba: The paralinguistic and linguistic conventions of the oral practice *chismeando*. *Research on Language and Social Interaction, 26*, 57-85.

Hall, J. K. (1993b). Oye, oye lo que ustedes no saben: Creativity, social power and politics in the oral practice of *chismeando*. *Journal of Linguistic Anthropology, 3*, 75-98.

Hannerz, U. (1967). Gossip, networks, and culture in a Black American ghetto. *Ethnos, 3*, 35-60.

Haviland, J. (1977). *Gossip, reputation and knowledge in Zinacantan*. Chicago: Chicago University Press.

Holmes, J. (1993). *Introduction to sociolinguistics*. London: Longman.

Hymes, D. (1974). *Foundations in sociolinguistics: An ethnographic approach*. Cambridge: Winthrop.

Lakoff, R. (1975). *Language and women's place*. New York: Harper & Row.

Morson, G., & Emerson, C. (1990). *Mikhail Bakhtin: Creation of a prosaics*. Stanford, CA: Stanford University Press.

Tolstoy, L. (1964). Why do men stupefy themselves? In *Leo Tolstoy: Selected essays* (A. Maude, Trans.). New York: Random House.

Vygotsky, L. S. (1978). *Mind in society: The development of higher psychological processes*. Cambridge, MA: Harvard University Press.

Wertsch, J. (1991), *Voices of the mind*. Cambridge, MA: Harvard University Press.

Wiarda, J., & Kryzanek, M. (1992). *The Dominican Republic: A Caribbean crucible*. Boulder, CO: Westview Press.

4

GENDER/LANGUAGE SUBTEXTS AS FOUND IN LITERATURE ANTHOLOGIES: MIXED MESSAGES, STEREOTYPES, SILENCE, ERASURE

MARY R. HARMON

Applebee (1993) found that nearly 66% of high school literature classes rely on anthologies as their primary source of literary selections and that over 88% of those teachers surveyed found these anthologies to be at least satisfactory in regard to the selections contained and the teaching apparatus included that accompany the heavy textbooks. (The Prentice Hall American literature text weighs in at more than 13 pounds!) Thus, the literature anthology plays a key role in U.S. high school literature classes. Authorized by the teacher, the classroom, the school, and sometimes state boards of education, anthologies, "embody the power to select (and therefore suppress), the power to shape and present certain aspects of human experience" (Scholes, 1985, p. 20). Through their content and form, contend Apple and Christian-Smith (1991), they "signify particular constructions of reality, particular ways of selecting and organizing that vast universe of possible knowledge" (p. 3). Anthologies, they continued, participate in the organized knowledge system of society and assist in "the creation of what a society has recognized as legitimate knowledge" (pp. 4-5; Apple, 1991).

Acknowledging the importance of high school literature anthologies, their selection as well as their nonselection materials (teaching apparatus), to the possible shaping or reinforcing of the thoughts and attitudes of a multitude of students, this chapter recounts my examination of the sociolinguistic texts and subtexts found in the most recent editions of five widely used high school U.S. literature anthologies' selections as well as their non-selection materials that comprise between 46% and 54% of their pages. I found that messages reinforcing dominant culture stereotypes and gender discrimination occur frequently in the choice of selections in all five anthologies, in their introductions of authors and selections, and in the questions and critical commentary they provide on selections, historical background, authors, and literary trends. In addition, these anthologies, all of which claim to offer students integrated approaches to language study, introduce little in the way of discussion and questions about the sociolinguistic aspects of language use, even when selections and critical commentary contain blatant examples of gender-biased language.

I examined the following five anthologies:

- *Adventures in American Literature* (1989). Pegasus Edition. Annotated Teacher's Edition. Harcourt Brace Jovanovich.
- *America Reads Series. The United States in Literature* (1991). Classic Edition. Teacher's Annotated Edition. Scott, Foresman.
- *Elements of Literature. Fifth Course. Literature of the United States* (1993). Annotated Teacher's Edition. Holt, Rinehart and Winston.
- *Literature and Language. Yellow Level. American Literature* (1992). Teacher's Annotated Edition. McDougal, Littell.
- *Prentice Hall Literature. The American Experience* (1991). Second Edition. Annotated Teacher's Edition. Prentice-Hall.

In the following, I consider and exemplify 10 means through which the anthologies examined in my study send students messages of gender bias and reinforce common gender stereotypes. Constraints of space and time prohibit my examples from being exhaustive lists; rather, they serve as illustrations of each of the 10 key points.

COVERS AND FRONTISPIECES

As soon as high school U.S. literature students receive their anthologies, a subtext of gender bias may begin working on them. Almost none of the anthologies studied depict either women or artifacts made by women on their front covers or in their frontispiece pictures. The possible exception is the frontispiece picture of the Statue of Liberty, a female in form if not in fact, draped by a quilt found in the McDougal Littell textbook. Prentice-Hall's cover and frontispiece both feature the portrait of Captain Joseph Reddeford Walker. Under his picture, every day, students and their teachers see the book's title, *The American Experience*. Inside the Teacher's Annotated edition, teachers are told that Walker, a White male trapper and adventurer represents the values of 19th century Americans (p. v). One is tempted to ask just whose experiences and values and which Americans this solitary White male does represent.

CONTENTS

The anthologies I studied all offer women limited representation and sometimes only token representation. Table 4.1 reports the number of female and male authors in the sample anthologies, the number of selections included in each textbook written by women and men, and the number of pages devoted to those selections. Numbers that appear to not "add up" correctly can be accounted for by anonymously written selections, several of which can be found in all the anthologies examined. As the table shows, the collections seriously under represent women. The highest percent of female authors is just over one in four (26.9%). The pages on which readers find selections written by women is even lower in all but one case. Prentice-Hall and Harcourt Brace Jovanovich offer only token representation (17% and 14%, respectively). The highest proportion of pages is one in three. What the numbers alone do not show is that the majority of selections written by women appear late in the anthologies on a one poem apiece basis or in the nonfiction portion of the book, much of which teachers do not assign students to read (Applebee, 1993). Few multiple entries or short works of fiction by women appear, and as Table 4.2 reveals, fewer long works (plays or full-length novels) written by women can be found. The numbers in Table 4.1 also fail to show that often the total pages of a few White male authors such as Whitman, Miller, Melville, Poe, Hawthorne, Emerson, Wilder, or Thoreau exceed all pages in the book written by women.

Table 4.1. Authors, Selections, and Pages.

Authors	Women (%)	Men (%)
PH-128	29 (22.7)	91 (71.1)
HBJ-134	24 (18)	105 (78.4)
SF-164	42 (25.6)	107 (65.2)
HRW-112	29 (25.9)	77 (68.8)
ML-93	25 (26.9)	64 (68.8)
Selections	Women (%)	Men (%)
PH-204	50 (24.5)	146 (71.6)
HBJ-233	46 (19.9)	182 (78.1)
SF-221	70 (31.6)	141 (64.3)
HRW-188	47 (25)	135 (71.8)
ML-108	28 (25.9)	76 (72.2)
Pages	Women (%)	Men (%)
PH-618	104 (16.8)	502 (81.2)
HBJ-575	78 (13.6)	493 (85.7)
SF-533	115 (21.6)	403 (75.6)
HRW-594	188 (24.9)	441 (74.4)
ML-471	156 (33.1)	308 (65.4)

Table 4.2. Long Works by Women and Men.

	Long Works	Women	Men
PH	1	0	1
HBJ	2	2	2
SF	2	0	2
HRW	2	1	1
ML	1	1	0

INTRODUCTIONS AND ESSENTIALIST STATEMENTS

With the exception of McDougal Littell, introductions to authors and their works appear before the works in the sample anthologies. Thus, students' and their teachers' readings of the works are likely influenced by the content and form of those introductions. In all five anthologies, White men tend are given longer introductions than other authors and, in cases where pictures are present, they have pictures included with the introductions. In two of the five examined anthologies, there was a pronounced difference in how female and male authors are introduced. As Table 4.3 reveals, Holt, Rinehart and Winston and Prentice-Hall introduce women more often in terms of their male mentors or family connections and the places in which they lived and men more often in terms of their literary accomplishments. Thus, repeatedly throughout these textbooks, students are transmitted messages that say achievement lies within the province of males.

The introductions of some women writers contain essentialist statements that lump together the works of all women and all minorities, thus diminishing the importance of individual writers and allowing for token representation of many diverse peoples by a few. Harcourt Brace places a heavy burden on Gwendolyn Brooks who is said to present both the African-American and the women's point of view. Note the use of the essentialist "the." To speak for all those peoples, Brooks is given two selection pages. Holt places an even heavier burden on Maxine Hong Kingston who, according to Holt, "speaks for some of the long stifled voices of Women, Native Americans, Blacks and other ethnic groups [note her own is not even mentioned], blue collar workers, and the poor, who did not in anthologies of the past often have the chance to tell their stories *directly*" (p. 1025, italics added). Ironically enough, Kingston does all of this in a short selection entitled, "The Girl Who Would Not Talk."

THEMATIC TOPICS OR ARRANGEMENTS

The thematic arrangements and topics suggested by four of the five anthologies bear out Jay's (1991) contention that thematic approaches are most often androcentric and "especially discriminatory . . . present[ing] a partial experience in the form of an eternal verity" (p. 211). With the exception of McDougal Littell, when anthologies offered thematic arrangements or included critical commentary on recurrent literary themes, the themes adopted largely excluded women writers and women's experiences. For example, as Scott, Foresman discusses the

Table 4.3. Modes of Introduction.

Accomplishments		Place	Other	People	Style
HRW	Women	7%	52%	28%	19%
	Men	49%	22%	13%	14%
PH	Women	40%	20.7%	21%	21%
	Men	81.3%	7.7%	4.4%	6.6%

theme of "Initiation," it names only 1 female but 12 male initiates. The "American Dream" theme includes only 1 female's but 11 male authors' works. The "Journey" theme features only 3 women travellers compared to 10 men. Harcourt Brace's section on "The American Novel" covers 33 novelists: 6 women and 27 men. Holt's "O Brave New World" theme lists 1 female-written and six male-written pieces; under "The Age of Reason" no women can be found; nor are there any under "The Individual and Society."

HISTORICAL BACKGROUND

All five anthologies introduce their literary units with historical background chapters. Table 4.4 shows how these chapters virtually erase the contributions of all but White males to the anthologies' versions of history. All of the anthologies' background chapters are accompanied by time lines, graphing chronologically the events covered in the chapters. As I looked at the events and the pictures included, I categorized them as female (Women's Rights Convention in Seneca, New York), male (World War II declared—women held few, if any, of the power positions that determined if and when the United States went to war), and neutral (San Francisco earthquake). In these versions of history, women play a very limited role. Does that matter? As early as 1979, Howe argued, "the images we pick up, consciously or unconsciously from literature and history significantly control our sense of identity and our identity" (p. 62). Gill (1993), professor of history at Yale Divinity School added, "The exclusion from history . . . has been women's most debilitating cultural deprivation. . . . Men's power to define what is political and what is not, what is historical and what is not, has left women adrift in an eternal present" (p. 12).

Table 4.4. Time-Line Events and Pictures.

	Women (%)	Men (%)	Neutral (%)
PH	33 (7)	431 (91)	10 (2)
HBJ	18 (8)	213 (92)	0
SF	33 (10)	281 (88)	4 (1.2)
HRW	30 (11)	235 (85)	12 (4)
ML	11 (7)	135 (88)	7 (4.6)
Time-Line Pictures			
PH	13 (11)	103 (86)	4 (3.3)
HBJ	5 (10.6)	32 (68)	5 (10.6)
SF	10 (23)	12 (28)	21 (49)
HRW	—	—	—
ML	3 (8.6)	19 (54)	13 (37)

GENDERED LANGUAGE, SEXIST LABELING, MISOGYNIST SELECTIONS

As Table 4.5 reveals, anthologies, despite their claims to integrated approaches, expend little space to discussions of sociolinguistic aspects of language use. When we remember that the typical anthology has more than 1,800 columns of space, the figures under each category in Table 4.5 demonstrate even more dramatically the scant attention paid to the sociolinguistic issues surrounding language use and users. Issues of sexist language are treated in especially limited fashion. Moreover, all five of these anthologies use sexist language themselves and fail to query such usage when it occurs in their selections. All contain a large number of pieces that use the term *girl* for adult women and which rely on the generic *he* and *man*. Despite all that has been written on the dismissal and exclusion inherent in such language use, not one of the anthologies addresses this issue in either critical commentary or the questions that follow selections. In fact, two of the anthologies (Scott, Foresman and Harcourt Brace), use the term *girl* to refer to adult women characters in selections by Henry James, Flannery O'Connor, and Dorothy Parker. Several of the anthologies use sexist labeling to refer to female characters in stories. Holt refers to Dame Van Winkle as an "ill-tempered shrew," and a "termagant" as well as a "nag." Rip, on the other hand symbolizes the "triumph of American innocence" (p. 121).

Table 4.5. Columns of Language Commentary and Questions.

	PH	HBJ	SF	HRW	ML
History					
• The changing nature of American English	4	13	16	39	1.5
Dialects					
• Definitions	.3	.3	.4	1.1	.5
• Dialects in American English	2.9	0	0	.6	3.8
• Authors' uses of dialect	1.4	6.4	.5	4	1.8
• Dialect as status/stigma	0	0	.06	.6	0
Registers					
• Standard English defined	0	0	0	0	.16
• Contrasts between standard and nonstandard forms; standard English grammar	20.5	.6	.2	102	152.7
• Language standards, setting standards, language control	.34	.4	.5	6.5	0
• formal, informal, slang forms	2.4	2	4.3	2.2	15
• Authors' uses of varied social registers	2	.5	2	6	1.2
• Status/stigma of varied registers	.8	.16	1.3	.2	2
Gender					
• The generic "he", "man"	0	0	0	0	0
• Authors' use of the above generics	0	0	0	0	0
• Other sexist language use	.16	.1	0	.06	.32
• Implications of sexist language use	0	.1	0	.06	.22
Ethnicity					
• Racist language use	.3	.2	0	.4	.7
• Implications of racist language use	.96	.5	0	0	.7
Names and Labels	3	.5	1	.44	1.04

Scott, Foresman uses similar terms to query Tom Walker's wife's actions and motives. In its Teacher's Notes, Holt describes Emily Dickinson as a spinster. McDougal Littell refers to the old, poverty stricken beggars in a Melville selection as "hags."

Even the most recently published anthology (the Holt anthology's 1993 edition), includes blatantly sexist labeling and commentary. About Anne Bradstreet, the introductory material reads, "Who would guess that the poet who would begin our literature would be an immigrant, teen-aged bride?" (p. 42). That Anne Bradstreet was 38, long married, and a colonial resident for a long period of time when her first work was published seems not to deter Holt as its labeling diminishes both Bradstreet and her work. As Holt comments on Emily Dickinson, students and their teachers are told that at first her life seemed "normal." "No one doubted that she would grow gracefully into womanhood, make a good marriage . . ." (p. 352). Thus, Holt narrowly defines the "normal" path for women. When Dickinson chose a less "normal" way of life, Holt describes her in terms of her dress and her marital state. She dressed "in white, like the bride she would never become" (p. 352) and died at the age of 56, "the perpetual bride who never crossed her own doorstep" (p. 353). Not until the last of a 4-column introduction does critical comment acknowledging Dickinson's achievements as a poet appear.

Scott, Foresman valorizes Hawthorne's assessment of the women writers of the 19th century as a "mob of scribbling women" by quoting it without examination. In fact, Scott, Foresman "elevates"only Harriet Beacher Stowe "above Hawthorne's ranks of scribbling women" (p. 265). Who judges literature and what is at stake in such judgements is never addressed nor is the role that respected male writers and critics such as Hawthorne may have played in ensuring the silence of women's voices, their denigration as authors, and their limited representation in anthologies such as this one. One is reminded of Dale Spender's (1989) contention that "Men have been in charge of according value to literature, and they have found the contributions of their own sex immeasurably superior" (p.1). Scott, Foresman again valorizes misogynist material when it quotes Nathaniel Ward's "humorous" lines depicting women and trouble as synonymous. No "humorous" lines critiquing men's behavior are quoted anywhere in Scott, Foresman.

Finally, because Scott Foresman fails to examine the sociolinguistic implications of the language use or the story itself, the inclusion of Harry Mark Petrakis' "The Wooing of Ariadne" must be discussed. The story features a male protagonist who has fallen in "love at first sight" with the beautiful and spirited Ariadne who consistently and emphatically refuses to speak to him or to see him. He launches a loud campaign to break down her opposition to him and harasses her at a dance, follows her, shouts to her from the sidewalk, talks to her priest after following her to church where he again creates a scene by shouting entreaties to her. She, the fulfillment of male fantasy, finally decides to see him and allow him to call on her, much to his triumph and joy. In the days of stalking laws and "no" means "no," the inclusion of this story by Scott, Foresman seems irresponsible as it teaches that sexual harassment will prevail and is a valid means of gaining one's will even as it teaches that women do not know their own minds. Rather than query the sociolinguistics of courtship and harassment, Scott, Foresman pronounces the male protagonist's final speech in the story as "eloquent" (p. 657). Thus, the anthology sends unexamined messages that stalking is legitimate, as in sexual harassment.

What, then are the messages students receive from their textbooks in regard to women, their expertise, their significance, their achievements, and their relationships to men? Women's works are insignificant, they belong at the back of the book. Women are virtually erased. Although they may write a short poem or two or an essay, the anthologies suggest women do not produce long works or serious works of fiction worth reproducing for a national audience. Women seem to play little or no role in the construction of United States' history. One or two women writers are sufficient to speak for all as well as for all minority persons. Women writer's lives and achievements are of interest primarily in regard to where they lived or which males they knew or were related to. Angry women are shrews, hags, nags, and termagants; others are "girls." Unmarried women are tragic "spinsters"; women's lives are normal only if they become men's "brides." Underlying all five of the anthologies is a strong subtext of the normalcy and necessity of heterosexual relationships; all five maintain absolute silence on homosexuality or homosexual relationships.

What can be done? As parents, teachers, and interested persons we can demand that schools and textbook publishers provide students with texts which do not promote and reinforce damaging sexist messages and stereotypes. As teachers and teacher educators, we can assist students in the critique of textbooks to alert them to the sexist messages they contain. We can deconstruct, defuse, and undermine the sexism of the anthologies through discussions of their inaccuracy and of who and how such messages benefit and damage. Apple (1991) reminded his readers that for the most part "hegemonic forms are not imposed from outside by small groups of corporate owners plotting how to do in workers, women, and people of color. . . . Dominant relations are reconstituted on an ongoing basis by the actions we take and the decisions we make in our own local and small areas of life" (pp.

34-35). Thus, as teachers and teacher educators, rather than participate in the skewed and damaging versions of literature and history as presented in the high school literature anthologies, we can assist students to construct alternative and oppositional versions, versions that empower women rather than relegate women (more than half the readers) to the back of the book.

REFERENCES

Apple, M. W. (1991). The culture and commerce of the textbook. In M. W. Apple & L. K. Christian-Smith (Eds.), *The politics of the textbook* (pp. 22-40). New York: Routledge & Kegan Paul.

Apple, M. W., & Christian-Smith, L. K. (Eds.). (1991). *The politics of the textbook.* New York: Routledge & Kegan Paul.

Applebee, A. N. (1993). *Literature in the secondary school.* Urbana, IL: National Council of Teachers of English.

Gill, K. (1993, May 2). A review of Gerda Lerner's the creation of the feminist consciousness. *The New York Times Book Review,* p. 12.

Howe, F. (1979). Sexual stereotypes start early. In P. Rose (Ed.), *Socialization and the life cycle* (pp. 52-63). New York: St. Martin's Press.

Jay, G. S. (1991, March). The end of "American" literature: Toward a multicultural practice. *College English, 53,* 264-281.

Scholes, R. (1985). *Textual power: Literary theory and the teaching of English.* New Haven, CT: Yale University Press.

Spender, D. (1989). *The writing or the sex.* New York: Pergamon.

Thompson, E., Bowler, E., Fried, P., Jackson, D., McCollum, D., Standen, J., Hickox, R., Schneider, C., & Ackley, K. (Eds.). (1991). *Prentice Hall literature. The American experience. Annotated teachers edition.* Englewood Cliffs, NJ: Prentice-Hall.

5

I NEVER TOLD ANYBODY AND I DESPERATELY NEED SOMEONE TO TALK TO: PROBLEM PAGES FOR GIRLS— RESEARCH ON ITALIAN TEEN MAGAZINES

PAOLA TRAVERSO

Publications aimed at teenage girls are growing in popularity in Italy. These magazines consist of features on romantic concerns, news and gossip about pop stars, regular articles on beauty and fashion, and sections for problem pages or advice columns.

These correspondence sections, where readers' problems are collected and answered, can be considered, in a certain sense, the core of the magazines. In these columns, the communication with the audience becomes more direct and intimate. It is here that the editors' intents become more evident. Promoting feminine culture, providing advice and instructions, offering psychological support and reassurance are, in fact, well integrated into these pages.

The main concern of the research presented here is to analyze which models of femininity these pages present to teenage girls and to investigate how messages are conveyed by both the selection of specific contents and the use of specific linguistic and journalistic techniques.

My particular interest in teen magazines, and in the models of femininity they provide, is dictated by the fact that puberty, more than any other period of life, signals the passage into womanhood and manhood. It is at this stage that learning how to act, behave, and speak according to one's own gender becomes particularly important. Young readers, because they are in a crucial stage of their sexual and social identity, are supposed to be particularly sensitive to any message on the female role, including those transmitted by the media.

The fact that the media play a part in the early socialization of children and in the long-term socialization of youth and adults is widely recognized. Various studies have been carried out on the issue of media and sex roles. Data have been collected on the diverse representation of the sexes (Butler & Paisley, 1980; Wartella, Whitney, & Windhall, 1983) and attention has been paid to the organization and production of culture and to the construction of an ideology of gender. (Daly, 1978; Tuchman, 1978).

In the past decades, women's magazines, even though less studied compared to other kinds of media, have yet provoked the interest of some scholars. Images of women in female journals have been examined and consequences of such representations have been discussed.

In the early 1960s, Betty Friedan (1963) pointed out the "Feminine Mystique" conveyed by women's magazines. More recent U.S. and British research (Ferguson, 1983; Hudson, 1984; Kramarae, 1981; McRobbie, 1982; Walkerdine, 1984) has stressed how these publications supply one source of definition of and socialization into the female role. They define and shape the woman's world, spanning every stage from childhood to old age.

FEMALE JOURNALS AND SEX ROLES:
THE ITALIAN PERSPECTIVE

In Italy, the interest in women's magazines as a social phenomenon goes back to the late 1950s. In 1959, Gabriella Parca published a book that caused a sensation. The volume, which was titled *Le Italiane si confessano*

(*Italian Women Confess*), was a collection of 8,000 letters that had appeared in female journals between 1955 and 1958.

The letters were grouped in several sections according to content, even though a single theme ran through the whole book: love and its troubles. From the pages, in fact, the image of unhappy and lonely women clearly emerged: housewives married to unfaithful men and suffering in silence; unfaithful housewives consumed with a sense of guilt; crying fiancées because "he " had broken off the engagement; girls attracted by married men and dreaming of impossible love; young teenagers in tears because they had not found a boyfriend.

In the introduction of the book, the author stated that the letters could be considered a mirror of what was happening in Italian society at the time—a mirror that reflected a submerged reality. According to Parca, in fact, these were things that women did not dare tell their mothers, their fiancées, their husbands; things that were taboo in the family were confessed in the problem pages. Although many would dissent with what Parca wrote, the book still remains an interesting document in the late 1990s.

In 1975, Buonanno published *Naturale come sei* (*As Natural as You Are*). The volume included a brief history of Italian magazines and a content analysis of those of the time. The author pointed out that modern female journals, as the ones first launched in the early 1920s, still focused on romance, fashion, house, family, and motherhood. An evolution had also taken place. Themes had broadened and some social issues had appeared: modern education for children, employment for women, divorce, sexual issues. Nevertheless, as Buonanno stated, changes in women's magazines were never very radical. When a new issue appeared, there had already been so much talk about it, that it was not new any more. The evolution of female journals, she wrote, was a marker of change in the condition of women in society, but not all changes were considered, or they were considered quite late.

It is not surprising, then, to see that very few changes have come about in teen magazines. As some articles pointed out (Garroni, Neonato, & Pietroforte, 1986; Marvelli, 1988; Turnaturi, 1986), romance, sexual issues, and themes related to the sphere of the personal are still predominant. Montanari (cited in Garroni et al., 1986) even called girls' journals "the priestesses of love."

History often repeats itself. In the 1950s, Italian women confessed their troubled love lives to their favorite magazines. In the late 1990s, teenagers write to the "priestesses of love" for advice. In my research, I have been trying to answer the following questions: What do they write about? What do they ask for? What are the so popular priestesses made of? What language do they speak?

THE POPULAR TEEN PUBLICATIONS: *CIOÉ, DOLLY, DEBBY*

Teen magazines launched in Italy in the late 1970s are a flourishing market but not yet firmly defined. At the time I began my research, 11 journals were on the market and some of them were quite recent. Among the variety of publications for teenage girls, three weeklies were chosen for analysis on the basis of their circulation figures: *Cioé, Dolly,* and *Debby*. The first two (see appendix A) were the only magazines of this genre to be included in *Indagine sulla Stampa Periodica Italia* (ISPI), the national survey on Italian periodicals. *Debby* was not included in ISPI but, among the recent journals, it appeared to be the most longlasting.

The titles and front covers of these three publications communicate at first glance that their audience comprises female teenagers. The titles of the magazines *Dolly* and *Debby* are Americanized girl names. For subtitles they use: "*Dolly*, your best friend," "*Debby*, the weekly of the heart." The title of the magazine *Cioé* literally translated means "that is." This was a very common expression some years ago.

The main ingredients of the three journals include letters to the editors, advice columns, features on romantic concerns and sexual matters, readers' true stories, gossip and activities of pop stars, quizzes to discover "what kind of girl you are," and some pages on beauty and fashion.

Correspondence sections occupy a large space. These deal with romantic concerns, sex, beauty, fitness and health, astrology and personality, interpretation of dreams and information about pop stars. However, not all of these appear in every issue. The regular and predominant ones are on romantic concerns and it is these columns that I examined.

ORGANIZATION OF THE STUDY

The three journals chosen for analysis, *Cioé, Dolly,* and *Debby,* have been examined over the period 1986 to 1989.

Twenty-four issues were collected for each magazine, selected during different seasons of the year to better assess changes attributable to the time of year. Twelve issues were collected during the 1986 to 1987 period and 12 during 1989 (see Appendix B).

Starting with the premise that content is as significant as form in putting the message across, the following points have been examined:

1. Content of the letters.
2. Journalistic techniques used in the columns.
3. Linguistic and communicative strategies used both in asking for and giving of advice.

ANALYSIS OF THE PROBLEM PAGES

"Any problem with your boyfriend, with your friends, with mom or dad? Don't know what to do? It's simple! Write to your best friend. She is waiting for you and she'll answer you!"

This is how the magazine *Dolly*, in its most important advice column named "Dear Dolly," invites young readers to write for any kind of advice. But what are the main questions the girls submit to the problem pages of their favorite journals? What are the main issues selected and published?

Agenda-setting is a common feature of the media. As McCombs and Shaw (1972) noted, editors and publishers decide what to place before the audience, they select issues, they set the order of priorities. It is possible to assume then, that the letters published in teen magazines are not a mere reflection of the girls' concerns, but are a reflection of the editors' agenda-setting of the feminine teenage world. They probably select the readers' letters in order of certain priorities; they may modify some of the letters published; they may even make up some of them.

My point is not to verify how many of the letters are real or how much they reflect a girl's world today. My intent is to examine the images of femininity that emerge from such pages.

In order to reach this goal, the letters have been classified according to their content. Six main subject matters have been pointed out: romantic concerns, sex, psychological issues, family, beauty, study and work. As Tables 5.1 and 5.2 show, the figure of the themes presented is quite similar for all three magazines. Most often mentioned are romantic concerns, but also there is a constant presence of psychological issues and of matters dealing with family and sex. Finally, a very small percentage of the letters deal with study and work. The last two subjects never appeared in *Cioé* and *Debby* until after 1987.

Certainly love, with its joy and excitement, anxiety and trouble, is the core of the letters. The girls write and ask how to get a boyfriend, what to do on a date, how to recognize a true love, how to cope with an impossible love, and how to survive love disappointments.

But the readers also express doubts, worries, and curiosities on sexual issues. They ask how to kiss and how to pet. They inquire about birth control methods. They worry about periods that have come too

Table 5.1. Dominant Themes, 1986 to 1987.

	Dolly (%)	Cioé (%)	Debby (%)	Total (%)
Romantic concerns	54.1	47.4	55.2	52.6
Psychological issues	13.8	13.5	18.4	15.4
Sex	8.3	11.8	17.1	12.5
Family	13.8	18.6	3.9	11.5
Beauty	0.3	—	2.6	3.8
Study and work*	—	—	—	—
Other	1.3	8.4	2.6	3.8
Total number of letters	72	59	76	207

*Specialized problem pages on study and work appear in the 1986-1987 period in four issues of Dolly.

Table 5.2. Dominant Themes, 1989.

	Dolly (%)	Cioé (%)	Debby (%)	Total (%)
Romantic concerns	43.3	50.9	50.9	46.6
Psychological issues	20.7	15.6	11.7	19.7
Sex	7.5	5.8	16.6	11.0
Family	13.2	17.6	4.9	10.0
Beauty	3.7	5.8	8.8	6.2
Study and work	7.5	1.9	1.9	3.3
Other	3.7	1.9	4.9	2.8
Total number of letters	53	51	102	208

early or that have not yet come, or about breasts that are too small or too large. They describe worries and fantasies related to masturbation and disappointment in sexual intercourse.

They complain of their unsatisfactory physical appearance. They ask for advice on overcoming shyness or solving conflicts with classmates or best friends. They say they are in trouble with strict parents who do not give them enough freedom: to wear make-up and clothes they like or to go out with friends and boyfriends.

There is a whole range of typical and stereotypical problems of adolescence, but certainly not an exhaustive range: love, emotions, interpersonal relationships, sex, personality, and physical appearance. The girls' concerns do not seem to go beyond this. Work and study are just occasionally mentioned. Sex is spoken about but nothing is said of the social relations of sexuality. Other possible social issues are ignored or dismissed. In the letters examined, for example, only one dealt with pornography and two with drug addiction. The world painted in the problem pages of these magazines is a world of "romance," timeless and classless. The readers seem to share the common, universal feminine teenage problems and to be united by a quest for advice on the arts and skills of femininity.

HOW TO BE THE GIRLS' BEST FRIEND: A QUESTION OF STYLE

Teen magazines, in their problem pages, claim to be the readers' confidant. To show that they are not pedant advisers but just good friends, they adapt a colloquial and informal style and they very often use an intimate tone.

Familiar and affectionate expressions are used by both sides. The letters open with Dear *Cioé*, Dear *Dolly*, Dear *Debby* and often end with regards and kisses. The girls very frequently sign with a diminutive related to the magazine title (a Dollina, a Debbina, a Cioé fan). Also in the replies the girls are addressed by such diminutives, to stress one more time the sense of belonging and membership among the female readers of that particular magazine.

The second-person singular pronoun "you" is the term of address most frequently used. It seems, in fact, quite suitable for an intimate one-to-one communication with the readers. However, in the replies expressions like "we," "we girls," "we all," "let's . . . ," "why don't we . . . ," also appear. This emphasizes a sense of togetherness and sisterhood, while at the same time denoting that the message is personal although it is for "all we girls."

A "write-to-speak" language is used both in the letters and in the replies. Verbs like "tell," "talk," are very frequent:

"I never told anybody and I desperately need someone to talk to."
"Dear Debbina, don't worry! I want to tell you that . . . !"

Feelings and emotions, very often present in the letters, are emphasized through the selection of certain verbs and adjectives. Girls do not just love, or like, or dislike. They are "madly in love," "crazy for him," they have "a super crush," or "they hate deeply," "they are so desperate!"

Slang expressions are very common. Teens use them especially when they need to refer to situations like falling in love, courting, flirting, and petting. The selection includes the most common and widely known phrases. They are seldom negative or vulgar; words with possible geographical connotations are carefully avoided. The same slang expressions may be reused in the replies, to keep a continuity of style with the readers and to give the impression that the dialogue is really from one friend to another who speaks the same language.

Proverbs sometimes appear in the replies. We find phrases like "If they are roses they will blossom," "Crying over spilled milk is not worth it." They recall old popular beliefs and values. They have familiarity because they are sayings the readers have already heard; they are common and collective knowledge that is handed from one generation to the next.

Even though the tone that pervades the problem pages is colloquial, familiar, and intimate, it is worth noting that the process of personalizing remains at a surface level. It seems as if two opposite tendencies are working at the same time: On the one hand, contents are personalized, whereas at the same time they are depersonalized. Issues presented in the letters are personal enough to appear authentic and real, but also at the same time general enough to interest a wide range of readers.

The girls who write are all Dolline, Debbine, Cioé fans and they are more often addressed with such diminutives than with their first names. Their age is almost always cited, whereas nothing is cited, at any rate, that could indicate their socioeconomic status. There is no mention of the kind of school they attend or, if they already work, of the kind of job they have. The facts presented in the letters published never specify biography or social contexts. They are just facts that happened to a Dollina, a Debbina, a Cioé fan and that could happen to any Dollina, Debbina, or Cioé fan.

ADVICE: ASKING AND RECEIVING

The main reason for the existence of the problem pages is, of course, the asking for and the receiving of advice. The communicative and linguistic strategies the readers use to express their problems are examined here, as well as the strategies used in the replies.

Asking for Advice

The majority of the letters published express problems, doubts, worries on romantic concerns and contain direct and explicit requests for advice, formulated through the use of different communicative and linguistic strategies (see Table 5.3). These requests are very often accompanied, on the one hand, by sentences of despair and on the other by declarations of confidence in the magazine like "Dear Debby, I have a terrible problem and I'm desperate. Help me, you are the only one I can confide in!" However, it appears that girls' attitudes and requests for advice are never totally passive. In fact, they may write "Help me!" "I need your advice," "What should I do?" "I do not know what to do any more," but they also make other requests.

They ask for a means to solve a certain problem because they want to succeed in their goals: "How can I do . . . ?" "Is there any way to . . . ?" They ask how to solve a dilemma, but they also elaborate on solutions they don't like: "Should I do this . . . or not do this?" "Don't tell me to. . . ." They may already have an idea of what to do in certain situations, including which decisions to make and write to the magazines just for reassurance and approval: "This story is absurd and I think if I break up with him once and for all it's better. What do you think? Loving dollina" (*Dolly*, 24 July 1989, p. 4).

Asking for help and advice, solution methods, instructions, and reassurance on how to cope with various romantic concerns are not the only points of the letters. The girls sometimes ask for explanations and help to better understand their own and other people's behavior and personality.

The presence of such requests is not a surprise. Being sensitive to feelings and emotions, taking care of other people's feelings and emotions are in fact feminine qualities girls and women are supposed to display. In some letters we find, therefore, sentences like: "What's happening to me?" "What does it mean?" "Why is he behaving like that?" "What does it mean?".

The readers not only ask for advice to better understand a certain behavior, they also express, in question form, their own hypotheses on the cases they are submitting and write "Maybe it is for this reason that . . . or maybe . . . ?" like in the following letter:

> Dear *Dolly*, I'm 14 and I'm in love with a boy of 20. When he sees me, sometimes he smiles at me and I don't know what to think. Is he in love as well maybe? Or is he too old for me and he just likes me? Susy (*Dolly*, 15 September 1986, p. 2)

Table 5.3. Advice Requests.

Linguistic Strategies

1. General Requests

Asking for help:	Help me! I need your advice.
Asking for advice:	I need your advice. Please give me your advice.
Asking what to do:	What should I do? What do you suggest that I do? I don't know what to do anymore. Tell me what to do.

2. Specific Requests

Asking for solution methods and instructions

Asking to solve a dilemma:	Should I do this . . . or not do this?
Asking for a means to:	How can I do . . . ? Is there any way to . . . ?
Stressing the unwanted solution:	Don't tell me to . . .

Asking help to understand their own behavior and personality

Asking for explanations:	What's happening to me? What does it mean?
Making hypotheses:	Maybe the reason is that . . . or maybe. . . ?

Asking help to understand other people's behavior and personality

Asking for explanations:	Why is she or he behaving like that? What does it mean?
Making hypotheses:	Maybe it is for this reason that . . . or maybe . . . ?

In conclusion, an active attitude seems to emerge from the letters. Teens write not only for general advice but to make specific requests, ask for specific solutions, express their own ideas, and formulate their own hypotheses. On the other hand, the kind of advice they are seeking involves traditional feminine topics: how to attract a boy, how to improve seduction, how to manage interpersonal relationships, how to better understand feelings and behaviors. The teen image that appears in the letters is one of active girls but also of girls who are deeply tied to the "feminine realm" of feelings and emotions and who want to be successful only in the tasks of femininity.

Giving Advice

Giving advice is the main goal of the problem pages. The tactics used to fulfill this task may be various and involve different linguistic and communicative strategies (see Table 5.4).

The analysis of the replies shows that advice is very often given in the form of suggestions, discussion about the problem, and expression of personal opinions like "Have you ever tried to . . . ?" "Why don't you . . . ?" "In my opinion . . ." "Maybe you are . . ." "Why do you . . . ?" "Don't you think that . . . ?". In a certain sense, it couldn't be different because in the letters the requests for help are not passive. As already noted, the girls who write to magazines very often express their ideas and hypotheses on the problem, they already know what a solution might be, or they have already tried one. On the other hand, because the problem pages claim to be the girls' best friend, an intimate and companionable tone seems more adequate than an authoritative one and more suitable to secure the readers' confidence.

Imperative forms are used just in special situations, where there is the necessity to exhort the reader to take a firm decision or to take an action.

> Break off at once, dear Patty. Such a guy doesn't deserve you. If he is behaving like that, it means he doesn't love you at all . . . (*Debby*, 9 March 1989, p. 2)

Imperatives are also used in step-by-step instructions, when advice needs to be given on how to improve physical appearance or personality aspects, like self-confidence or self-determination. But, in the majority of cases, suggestions are preferred to step-by-step instructions with imperatives.

Another important aspect of the replies is that advice is usually given using a personal tone (use of second-person pronoun "you," of first names of the readers or of affectionate appelatives). When remarks are directed to all the readers, they are often invitations to do something or to change an attitude: "Let's do this!" "Why don't we . . . ?" Such sentences, besides stressing a sense of commonality and membership using the pronoun "we," underline the importance of active doing and of self-determination.

In addition, readers are reassured about their doubts and anxieties and they are told not to worry because certain reactions are normal, that there is a solution to their problems and, most important of all, that they can make it:

Table 5.4. Giving Advice.

Linguistic Strategies	
1. Advising What to Do	
Directives constructed as suggestions:	Try to . . . Have you ever tried to . . . ? Why don't you . . . ?
Directives constructed with the imperative:	Do this!
Step-by-step instructions constructed with the imperative:	Do this and this. Then . . .
Advice stated as personal opinion:	I think the best thing to do is . . .
2. Helping to Understand Personality and Interpersonal Relationships	
Stating what the problem is:	Your problem is . . . You are . . .
Stating what the problem is using the form of personal opinion:	I think your problem is . . . In my opinion . . .
Suggesting explanations:	Maybe you are . . . Maybe he is . . .
Stimulating by questions:	Why do you . . . ? Don't you think that . . . ?
3. Advice Directed to All the Readers	
Invitations:	Let's do this! Why don't we do . . . ?
Stimulation by questions:	Why do we . . . ? Why do you . . . ?

"You'll see that everything turns out for the best."
"You'll see that you are able to do that."
"You'll see that you feel better."
"You'll see that is not so difficult as it looks."

CONCLUSION

The analysis of the problem pages of *Cioé*, *Dolly*, and *Debby* has shown the prevalence of a discourse centered on the sphere of the personal: love, sex, emotions, and interpersonal relationships. A sphere that does not seem to be threatened by any social conflicts at all.

If content is carefully selected, on the other hand, language is shaped and selected as well. Hyperboles are common for describing feelings; slang is used but it cannot be too vulgar; colloquialism and informal style are the rule because the "talk" must appear to take place between friends.

The results of my research are not very different from those of some U.S. and British studies on women and teen magazines already cited (Ferguson, 1983; Hudson, 1984; Kramarae, 1981, McRobbie, 1982). The authors have widely pointed out the role of these publications in maintaining and promoting the cult of femininity. In fact, even though longitudinal analyses have shown that these publications are not completely insensitive to changes that are happening in society, the cult of femininity remains their main goal.

As has already been noted, the Italian sociologist Buonanno (1975) stressed that nevertheless social changes maybe registered in these publications, they appear only partially and later than reflected in real life.

These considerations seem to apply also to the teen magazines I have examined. In fact, they remain deeply centered in the sphere of the personal, even though they reveal some innovations in the way of looking at certain issues and in the way of the asking for and the giving of advice.

For example, getting a boyfriend is still a primary goal. But, although in the past it meant the steady boyfriend or the future spouse, here the emphasis is on improving relationships with the opposite sex and seductive capabilities in general.

Sex is spoken about quite frequently because, with changes in social mores that have taken place since the 1960s, certain topics, like contraception or extramarital sex, are no longer considered taboo, even for young adolescents. However, social relations of sexuality are not discussed, nor are other issues like sexual harassment, rape, or pornography.

In asking for advice, the letters published give the image of teens who trust and deeply confide in their favorite magazines. But this does not mean that the girls are waiting passively for the magic answer. In many cases, they express their ideas and hypotheses on the problem and may even anticipate possible solutions.

In the replies, advice is offered, but the tone is not directive and suggestions are offered in a friendly and companionable style. This seems more suitable to today's girls who live in a society less authoritarian and repressive than the past and who have a wider range of experiences and opportunities, like studying, working and traveling.

Society changes, adolescents change and female journals must change, too. But they try to do it as little as possible. As a matter of fact, in these magazines the traditional feminine qualities of being attractive, seductive, sensitive to feelings and emotions are still pictured as the desirable qualities for a girl. Also, self-confidence and self-determination are viewed as important and desirable but, alas, they just apply to sentimental matters. In fact, besides romantic concerns other possible social issues are ignored or dismissed. The discourse remains centered on the secrets and skills of femininity, an art to be passed from one generation to the next.

Table A.1. Teenage Girl Publications Market

Name of the Magazine	Editors	Year	Genre
Sì	Edifumetto	1987	Weekly
Cioé	Cioé srl	1979	Weekly
Dolly	Mondadori	1977	Weekly
Pupa	Cioé srl	1987	Weekly
Rosa Shocking	Play Press	1987	Fortnightly
Debby	Cioé srl	1986	Weekly
Segreti	Play Press	1987	Monthly
Hallo	Leti srl	1986	Weekly
Astrella	Cioé srl	1987	Monthly
Cleò	Cioé srl	1987	Weekly
Be Bop A Ula	Edifumeto	1986	monthly

Note. Data published in Città Nuova (No. 5 1988)

Table A.2. Circulation Data.

	1986	1987	1989
Cioé	213,628	272,855	273,537
Dolly	198,279	133,638	115,935

Note. Data from ISPI (1986, 1987, 1989).

Table A.3. Age Distribution of Readers.

Age	Cioé (%)	Dolly (%)
14-17	49.3	42.2
18-24	22.2	33.2
25-35	9.2	12
35-44	12.3	5.5
45-54	5	3.6
55-64	.9	2.7
64+	1.1	.9
Total	100	100

Note. Data from ISPI (1989).

Table A.4. Social Class Distribution of Readers.

Social Class	*Cioé* (%)	*Dolly* (%)
A	12.8	13.3
B	35.4	40.7
C	18.1	15.5
D	29.8	27.3
E	3.9	3.2
Total	100	100

Note. A = high, B = middle high, C = middle, D = middle low, E = low.
Data from ISPI (1989).

Table B.1. Issues Examined.

Cioé

No 38,	21 September 1986	No 12,	20 March 1989
No 39,	28 September 1986	No 13,	27 March 1989
No 40,	5 October 1986	No 14,	10 April 1989
No 41,	12 October 1986	No 15,	17 April 1989
No 4,	19 January 1987	No 26,	3 July 1989
No 5,	26 January 1987	No 27,	10 July 1989
No 6,	2 February 1987	No 28,	17 July 1989
No 7,	9 February 1987	No 29,	24 July 1989
No 28,	6 July 1987	No 39,	2 October 1989
No 29,	13 July 1987	No 40,	9 October 1989
No 30,	20 July 1987	No 41	16 October 1989
No 31,	27 July 1987	No 42,	23 October 1989

Dolly

No 413,	15 September 1986	No 545,	27 March 1989
No 414,	22 September 1986	No 546,	3 April 1989
No 415,	29 September 1986	No 547,	10 April 1989
No 416,	6 October 1986	No 548,	17 April 1989
No 432,	26 January 1987	No 560,	10 July 1989
No 433,	2 February 1987	No 561,	17 July 1989
No 434,	9 February 1987	No 562,	24 July 1989
No 435,	16 February 1987	No 563,	31 July 1989
No 456,	13 July 1987	No 573,	9 October 1989
No 457,	20 July 1987	No 574,	16 October 1989
No 458,	27 July 1987	No 575,	23 October 1989
No 459,	3 August 1987	No 576,	30 October 1989

Debby

No 27,	10 September 1986	No 41,	9 March 1989
No 28,	17 September 1986	No 42,	30 March 1989
No 29,	29 September 1986	No 43,	13 April 1989
No 30,	1 October 1986	No 44,	27 April 1989
No 4,	22 January 1897	No 48,	22 June 1989
No 5,	29 January 1987	No 49,	6 July 1989
No 6,	5 February 1987	No 50,	20 July 1989
No 7	12 February 1987	No 51,	3 August 1989
No 29,	16 July 1987	No 55,	28 September 1989
No 30,	23 July 1987	No 56,	12 October 1989
No 31 ,	30 July 1987	No 57,	26 October 1989
No 32,	6 August 1987	No 58,	9 November 1989

REFERENCES

Buonanno, M. (1975). *Naturale come sei* [As natural as you are]. Guaraldi Editore.

Butler, M., & Paisley, W. (1980). *Women and the mass media: Sourcebook for research and action.* New York: Human Sciences Press.

Daly, M. (1978). *Gyn/ecology: The metaethics of radical feminism.* Boston: Beacon Press.

Ferguson, M. (1983). *Forever feminine.* Brookfield, VT: Gower Publishing.

Friedan, B. (1963). *The feminine mystique.* New York: Dell.

Garroni, S., Neonato, S., & Pietroforte, S. (1986). *Parole incrociate* [Interlaced words]. Edizioni Cooperative Libera Stampa.

Hudson, B. (1984). Femininity and adolescence. In A. McRobbie & M. Nava (Eds.), *Gender and generation* (pp. 31-53). New York: Macmillan Education.

Kramarae, C. (1981). *Women and men speaking.* Rowley, MA: Newbury House.

Marvelli, G. (1988). Come ti erudisco il teen-ager [How to train teenagers]. *Citta Nuova* [New City], *5,* 34-37.

McCombs, M. E., & Shaw, D. L. (1972). The agenda-setting function of the press. *Public Opinion Quarterly, 36,* 176-187.

McRobbie, A. (1982). JACKIE: An ideology of adolescent femininity. In B. Waites, T. Bennett, & G. Martin (Eds.), *Popular culture: Past and present* (pp. 263-283). London: Croom Helm-The Open University Press.

Tuchman, G. (1978). The symbolic annihilation of women. In G. Tuchman, K. Daniels, & J. Benet (Eds.), *Hearth and home: Images of women in the mass media* (pp. 3-38). New York: Oxford University Press.

Turnaturi, G. (1986, April 6). Cara Dolly, come si fa l'amore? [Dear Dolly, can you tell me how to make love?]. *Espresso,* 83-85.

Walkerdine, V. (1984). Some day my prince will come. In A. McRobbie & M. Nava (Eds.), *Gender and generation* (pp. 162-184). New York: Macmillian Education.

Wartella, E., Whitney, D. C., & Windhall, S. (Eds.). (1983). *Mass communication review yearbook* (Vol. 4). Thousand Oaks, CA: Sage.

6

ROMANCING THE EARTH: FEMINIZED NATURE AND MATERNAL/EROTIC METAPHORS IN RECENT ECO-ENVIRONMENTAL LITERATURE

LENORA A. TIMM

Metaphors may create realities for us, especially social realities. A metaphor may thus be a guide for future action. Such actions will, of course, fit the metaphor. This will, in turn, reinforce the power of the metaphor to make experience coherent. In this sense metaphors can be self-fulfilling prophecies.
—Lakoff & Johnson (1980, p. 156)

Metaphor, simile, and personification are among the most useful communicative devices we have, because by their quick affective power they often make unnecessary the invention of new words for new things or new feelings.
—Hayakawa (cited in Kolodny, 1975, p. 149)

105

Metaphorical language and its influence on conceptualization has been the subject of scholarly ruminations in the West since the time of classical Greek civilization. Both Plato and Aristotle, for example, had a great deal to say about metaphors; Plato abjuring them on the grounds that they clouded or distorted pure thought, whereas Aristotle favored them as ornaments of speech that at the same time served to stimulate the mind by their puzzle or enigma like qualities. European writers of the Middle Ages were much given to allegories (i.e., extended metaphors) and the prose and poetry of the 19th-century Romantics are notable for their impassioned metaphoric imagery.

Yet it would be a mistake to think that metaphors dwell chiefly in high literature or classical erudition, for as research by scholars from many disciplines has shown, our everyday talk is studded with metaphorical turns of phrase, many of them so routinized in our speaking and writing habits that we scarcely recognize them as such (e.g., the eye of a needle, the mouth of a river, a hot topic, borrow an idea, etc.). Lakoff and Johnson (1980), for example, argued that metaphors serve as conceptual anchors for our perceptions and to some extent for our behaviors: They provide a means by which we understand the world around us, apprehend causality, make connections across disparate sets of objects or relations, and are a means through which we make evaluations. Schön (1979) characterized metaphor in two ways: First, as "a perspective or frame, a way of looking at things" and, second, as "a process by which new perspectives on the world come into existence" (p. 254). Yet, if it is true that metaphors help us see aspects of reality previously unseen or unperceived, it may also be the case that metaphors work to constrain or channel our vision, or lead us to see some features of a situation at the expense of others (Ortony, 1979). It is this particular potential of metaphors that is my focus here, for I am concerned with the "stories" told both about women and about nature and the earth by the female-related metaphors that have become so prevalent in discussions of the environment and the ecological health of the planet. I am concerned that the framing of environmental problems within a female-identified metaphor (a) leads us down a path of thought that forecloses other avenues we might travel to understand the human-nature relationship; and (b) continues to associate women with traditional roles and behaviors (as mother, nuturer, caretaker, and object of erotic allure). These matters are examined later. In the next section, I provide a brief background on scholarly research on metaphors.

HOW METAPHORS WORK

It was long maintained by linguists and philosophers (following Aristotle) that metaphors work by expressing a perceived similarity between or among things, people, animals, and so on. But this definition is quite limiting, and does not help account for even some of the most commonplace metaphors. More recent analyses of metaphor describe what it accomplishes in terms of the connections it invokes between domains (Sweetser, 1990), which may not have any perceptible similarity, but that, for a complex of sociocultural and psychosocial reasons, lead people to "see" something or someone or some process or event in a new light.[1] This approach to metaphor has been called *perspectival*, and it grows out of the work of philosopher Max Black (1962) and others over the past 25 to 30 years, notably linguist Eva Feder Kittay (1987), whose model of metaphor I lean on in my own analysis.

In discussing how a metaphor functions, from a perspectival approach, the convention has arisen of speaking of an interaction between that which is the subject or *topic* of the metaphor and that which is the *vehicle* of the metaphor.[2] Thus, in an example from some early Christian writings—*A woman is the Devil's gateway*—the topic of this metaphor is "woman" in a generic sense, and the vehicle used to represent something about this topic is, obviously, the gateway to the Devil, itself an allegorical way of representing evil. As Kittay pointed out (1988), "the choice of vehicle can itself reveal much about the way in which the topic is conceived" (p. 81) by the speaker (and by implication by the speaker's culture or social group). To pursue this thought, it is a striking fact about the vehicles of metaphor in English (and other European languages) that they are often derogatory or otherwise negative when the topic is related to women. And, conversely, a topic is often represented in negative terms by the vehicle, when the latter depicts a woman or female nature.[3] In addition, metaphors involving

---

[1]"Metaphor or, at least, metaphor shaped through the imagination, does not record pre-existing similarities in things; rather, it is the linguistic means by which we bring together and fuse into a unity diverse thoughts and thereby re-form our perceptions of the world. Symbols such as a national flag, a crest, and object with ritualistic significance . . . also involve such fusion" (Kittay, 1987, p. 6).

[2]The terms *vehicle* and *tenor* (for *topic*) were first introduced by Richards (1936).

[3]Both of these patterns are visible in many proverbs, aphorisms, and lines from well-known literary works. For example, in (i) through (iii) "woman" or one of her attributes is the topic of a derogatory proverb; in (iv) through (v) "woman" is the vehicle by which the topic is denigrated:

women are often sexually or erotically evocative.[4] With this background in mind, I move on to the specific metaphors with which I am concerned in this chapter (i.e., the earth-is-our-mother metaphor and the personification of nature as female). I argue that these essentially androcentric figures of speech pre-empt the metaphoric ground on which a female-based understanding of earth-human relations might be established

"MOTHER EARTH" THROUGH TIME

The metaphorization of earth reaches far back in time. The Greeks worshiped in their pantheon of deities Gaia, the Earth Mother, their oldest goddess, who has come to prominence in the West once again with the development within scientific circles of the so-called Gaia Hypothesis, to which I return in next section. The Homeric poems (c. 700 BC) were already rich in metaphoric maternal imagery, depicting a "wide-bosomed Earth, mother of gods and men, animals and plants. She nourishes and cares for all creatures as her own children" (Hughes, 1982, p. 94).[5]

The metaphoric association of maternal femaleness with the earth and nature in general was thus established early in the West. However, an important shift in the metaphor, documented by Merchant (1980) in *The Death of Nature*, accompanied the Baconian revolution in scientific methodology. That is, from nature envisaged as a benevolent,

---

(i) A wife's long tongue is the staircase by which misfortunes ascend to the house (Mieder, 1966).

(ii) A woman's tongue breaks bones (Mieder, 1966).

(iii) Woman is the lesser man (Tennyson).

(iv) Frailty, thy name is woman (Shakespeare).

(v) Fortune is a woman and it is necessary if you wish to master her to conquer her by force (Machiavelli, cited in Kittay, 1988, p. 72).

[4]Negative interpretations of women are grounded in millennia of misogynistic thinking and writings, from the Greeks through the early Christian theologians to the Middle Ages and up to present day. This history is not addressed here; some excellent sources for exploring it include Bloch (1991), Pagels (1988), Ruether (1974, 1983), and others.

[5]A look at various cultures across time and space reveals that the earth is often conceptualized as a maternal female; this is true, for example, of many Native American cultures (Weigle, 1989). There is compelling archaeological evidence, as well, from the Mediterranean area and southeastern Europe (Gimbutas, 1982, 1989) of the worship of powerful goddesses by societies that existed millennia ago; doubtless included among their ranks are earth goddesses.

caring mother, with whom humans existed in organic harmony, 17th to 18th century "Natura" came to be viewed as a willful and capricious female who must be subdued and controlled for the benefit of "mankind." Renowned for his advocacy of the empirical approach to science, Bacon argued that with proper methodology and techniques, Nature could be mastered and induced to deliver up her secrets.[6]

Writings from 17th century natural philosophers on the subject of nature thus began to travel another metaphoric path, drawing inspiration from two familiar masculine behaviors vis-à-vis women: domination and seduction. For these early scientists, when the topic is nature, the metaphorical vehicle is more often than not woman from a male perspective, and the theme of conquering and controlling nature is increasingly in evidence.[7]

For example, Bacon urged male scientists to join forces against nature "to storm and occupy her castles and strongholds" (Easlea, 1980, p. 248). Isaac Barrow (Newton's teacher) proclaimed that the mission of the new (mechanistic) philosophy was to "search Nature out of her concealments, and unfold her dark Mysteries." The historian of the Royal Society, Thomas Sprat, selected the seduction twist on nature imagery, arguing that nature "is also a Mistress" who will yield to the most ardent suitor; he was confident that the Royal Society's "Courtship to Nature would eventually expose her 'Beautiful Bosom' to the view and satiation of its members." Thomas Vaughan, an alchemist and philosopher, advocated coercion and rape, warning philosophers that they should on no account be content to "'lick the shell' of nature but must 'pierce . . . experimentally in the Center of things.' Well might Nature complain, continued Vaughan, that he had 'all most broken her Seale, and exposed her naked to the World'" (Easlea, 1980, p. 247).

Although these statements may strike the modern reader as arcane *exempla* of the rhetoric of a bygone age, data from recent sources demonstrate that the woman-nature/mother-earth affinities are still present in people's minds, doubtless especially in male minds, and may

---

[6]It has been claimed (Merchant, noted in Li, 1993, p. 277) that Bacon's new methodology drew on the interrogatory practices (including torture) applied to people suspected of being witches during this epoch, 90% of whom were women.

[7]In a recent study of the origins of modern science in medieval and early modern Europe, Famon (1994) stressed the salience of the metaphor of the hunt— "Science as a *Venatio*," is the title of one chapter—in the writings of the 17th-century philosophers. He pointed out that "the 'search for secrets' in unknown regions of nature was an image that appeared in the period's scientific literature with monotonous regularity" (p. 273). Remarkably, however, he nowhere even mentioned the sexual metaphors embedded in so many of the statements made by the Renaissance male investigators he discussed.

find expression in forms not far removed from those articulated in the 17 to 18th centuries. I refer especially to the renewal and intensification of female-identified nature in the wake of what has come to be called the Gaia Hypothesis, to which I turn now.

THE GAIA HYPOTHESIS

This scientific theory was first formulated by British atmospheric chemist James Lovelock and American microbiologist Lynn Margulis, and was made widely accessible to the public in Lovelock's (1979) paperback book, *Gaia, A New Look at Life on Earth*.[8] Briefly, Lovelock and Margulis argued that the the earth's surface environment, including temperature, climate, oxidation state, and acidity, is regulated by the interaction among the plants, animals and microorganisms that reside in it; that, further, the planet has—in some sense—a capacity to adjust and regulate itself to maintain homeostasis. In other words, earth may be said to constitute a colossal integrated organism, which, like any living being, is able to make adjustments to stress and trauma and, in effect, to heal itself over time. The hypothesis is controversial in that it flies in the face of traditional views of the earth as an inanimate globe, whose formation and evolution have been controlled principally by geological forces and not biological ones. Under the Gaian view, the earth is seen as more resilient and less fragile due to its hypothesized adaptability, than under the traditional earth sciences interpretation of planetary stability.[9]

---

[8]Novelist William Golding, a neighbor of Lovelock's in Cornwall is said to have suggested to him naming his theory "Gaia."

[9]Controversial as a hypothesis among scientists, Gaia has nonetheless enjoyed considerable success as a commercial venture, notably among New-Agers who for more than a decade have been marketing Gaia spirituality artwork, crafts, and self-help books. Private Gaia foundations and institutes have been established in the United States and in Europe; and the Commonwealth Institute of London created a new hymn to Mother Earth, "Gaia Song," which has been disseminated to the 49 countries of the British Commonwealth (in Joseph, 1990, p. 66):
Gaia is the one who gives us birth

> She's the air, she's the sea, she's Mother Earth
> She's the creatures that crawl and swim and fly,
> She's the growing grass, she's you and I.

The Love Your Mother! bumper sticker, commonly seen in the 1980s, is yet another instantiation of popular response to the the Earth Mother metaphor (Seager, 1993).

Pushing the metaphor further, Lovelock at one point intimated that Gaia, the earth, had a mind and will of its own, with intentionality; but Gaia's body was clearly imaged by him as female and the human scientist imaged as (a heterosexual) male.[10] This emerges in the final chapter of his 1979 book, in which he proposed to discuss "intangible aspects of the Gaia hypothesis: those which concern thought and emotion in the interrelationship of man and Gaia" (p. 141). He continued,

> Let us start by considering our sense of beauty . . . there seems no need inevitably to attribute the pleasure we feel on a country walk, as our gaze wanders over the downs, to our instinctive comparison of the smooth, rounded hills with the contours of a woman's breasts. The thought may indeed occur to us; but we could also explain our pleasure in Gaian terms. (p. 142)

Despite Lovelock's use of the first-person plural pronoun "we/our," the perspective expressed in this passage is indisputedly that of a heterosexual man, and the "interrelationship of man and Gaia" looks suspiciously like that of a horny male human lusting after a beautiful woman seen at a distance. In this passage coopting the human perspective by the specious invocation of "man" results in a singularly narrow and, it might be argued, deceptive and exclusionary vision of the human-earth relationship.[11]

The androcentric stance is commonplace. For instance, we find in the first paragraph of Sale's (1982) popular book, *Dwellers in the Land*, a description of earth as "a vibrant globe of green and blue and grey binding together in a holy, deep-breasted synchrony . . . a pulsing body . . . Gaia, the earth mother" (p. 3). In Tobias' (1990) recent popularization of the Gaia hypothesis in *Voice of the Planet*, a book later made into a 10-hour television series, Gaia (played by Faye Dunaway) is cast as a sexy, sultry, and mysterious female. She shamelessly flirts with the male hero, a handsome, blue-eyed, White ecologist (played by William Shattner), who has taken a year's leave from CalTech to write a book on the impact of humans on the planet; Mother Earth is his guide for the year. Gaia communicates with him through a computer that has been jimmied by a Tibetan monk to give a direct line to the ancient goddess. Much of the narrative as well as the dialogue between the main human character, William Hope Planter, and

---

[10]For the record, Margulis strongly repudiated the maternal imagery and ecotheological ruminations that have flowed from the theory (Joseph, 1990).

[11]For an excellent critical review of feminized Gaia imagery as found in the writings of deep ecologists and of some ecofeminists and ecopoets, see Murphy (1988).

Gaia slides uneasily back and forth between mother-child talk and sex talk, in a schizoid affirmation of Freudian oedipal psychoneurosis.[12]

Although Gaia in this bizarre fantasy is a principal character, her voice is one created and controlled by a male writer, and through it he projects his own psycho-sexual impulses. An authentic female voice and viewpoint on the human-earth relationship are not simply marginalized, they are absent, pre-empted by the irrepressible metaphorical imagery of a sex goddess/earth mother.

CRITIQUE OF THE EARTH AS MOTHER/SEX OBJECT METAPHOR

As I see it, two sets of problems emerge when the earth and nature are metaphorized as a female, whether maternal or sexually alluring in guise. The first set relates to the effect of such metaphors on ecological and environmental conceptualizing and strategizing; the second to the effect on what I term the epistemological and cultural status of women. I start with the former set of issues.

First, consider the bumper sticker that enjoins the observer to *Love Your Mother*, the metaphor for "earth." What images are the reader of this decal likely to conjure up? Presumably those corresponding to one of two fairly stereotypic perceptions of mothers in the society at large: (a) the idealized perception of a mother as kind, nurturing, giving, and forgiving; or (b) a contrasting perception of a mother as controlling, disapproving and judgmental. From an environmental point of view, however, the first perception is surmountingly naive, for there are no scientific grounds for believing that the natural forces on the earth are either "kind" or "nurturing" or that they will "forgive" humans their destructive ways and take care of them forever with an infinite cornucopia of resources. On the other hand, the second perception is more likely to conjure up the image of a vengeful Mother Nature, wrecking havoc with her hurricanes, droughts, or pestilences. It is not easy to love this sort of mother; one would be more inclined to seek

---

[12]For example, Planter described Gaia's voice as "rich in softness and wit, intelligence and the erotic" (Rose, 1993, p. 154). He wrote in his diary that the computer "monitor is bright blue, the mechanical love machine—her inner eye, like a piston enveloping itself in masturbatory rhythm—floods the room with sexual light" (Rose, 1993, p. 154). Gaia often orders Planter to "stroke me," supposedly a command to spin the prayer wheel attached to the computer. The erotic later dissolves into the maternal, as Gaia chides Planter for not eating enough; he retorts, "you're beginning to sound just like my mother" (Rose, 1993, p. 155. For a fuller discussion, see Rose, 1993).

ways—*à la* Francis Bacon—to control and constrain her. Indeed, one study of the imagery in pesticide ads finds, unsurprisingly, that agribusiness "sees nature as a force to be conquered," and for many years now has promoted a battery of products with such military names as Surefire, Colonel, TopGun, Marksman, Salute, Bladex, Scepter, Squadron, and Bayonnet (Ahlberg, 1988).[13] Such an approach to weed control is ecologically maladaptive; many researchers in the environmental sciences have come to realize that it is far more effective in the long run to work with natural biota—by striving to understand the intricate workings of biotic communities—rather than to seek only to exterminate by means of concocted poisons those deemed "undesirable."

Second, this society includes a strong tendency to devalue motherhood, at least to denigrate the real activities associated with motherhood—infant and child care, housework, chauffeuring children around, helping with homework, volunteering at schools, and so on. None of these activities is accorded high value by our society, certainly not as measured by monetary criteria. Will it prove helpful or, rather, defeating of one's good intentions vis-à-vis the environment to associate the earth with femaleness and/or with motherhood, both of which have had subordinate status throughout history and have arguably been more often denigrated than esteemed? As Garb (1990) said, "What baggage will carry over from one domain to another (especially in a culture whose relation to both women and mothers is as misogynous as ours is?" (p. 277).

The serious science that is being done on the Gaia Hypothesis[14] concludes that it is the colligative interaction among all the different biota and the inanimate parts of the planet that bring about the self-regulating homeostasis that make life sustainable. Such a process, or interaction, is very poorly metaphorized as a mother-child relationship. The earth is neither a powerful and bountiful mother nor a sexy goddess who will take care of "her" children if they are good and obedient and love her, or punish them if they misbehave and abuse her.[15] Rather, it seems far more likely, as the deep ecologists aver, and as the Gaia Hypothesis posits, that all components of the planet, from tiny microbes to soaring mountain tops, are involved (without intention as humans know it), in intense and ceaseless interaction. Within this

---

[13]Research by Ahlberg (1988), reported in G. Gaard (1993, p. 304).

[14]See, for example, Allaby (1990), Bunyard and Goldsmith (1989), Dyson (1992), Thompson (1987), Gribbin (1990), Schneider and Boston (1991).

[15]On the contrary, as Miller (1991, p. 2) observed: "it is today humankind that has the power to determine Gaia's future," not the other way around.

conceptualization of the earth, each element exerts an influence, however infinitesimal it may be, on the earth's environment. What metaphor might we invoke to capture this picture of interaction and of interrelationships among participants? At the moment, I do not have one, but I believe it would be a useful exercise if scientists working within the framework of the Gaia Hypotheses were to start thinking seriously about this question. The second set of objections raised above focus on the impact on women of the metaphorical linking of maternity with the earth and nature. This linkage and the existence of such slogans as Love Your Mother certainly reinforce the conceptual connection between human females and nature in general, and by implication distance them from culture, which in Western tradition has been strongly associated with human males. In fact, a great deal has been written on the alleged bond between women and nature, on the one hand, and men and culture, on the other. The problem with these associations has always been that the female-nature side has been judged as inferior to the male-culture side, because female-nature is considered less rational, less trustworthy, less active, less fully human, and often (ironically) less creative than the male/culture side.[16]

At the same time, an impulse within eco-feminism has—paradoxically it might be argued—not only acknowledged the woman/nature connection but endorsed and embraced it (Collard, 1989; Eisler, 1987; Griffin, 1978; LaChapelle, 1988; 1982; Spretnak, 1982). I believe that feminists, eco- and otherwise, should not unreservedly buy into this "essentialist" interpretation of women as somehow more natural than men. The proposed affinity implicitly sanctions the view of sex/gender roles as biologically determined, a belief that has brought great grief to women in the past, based on fallacious claims about woman's physical and mental limitations due to her reproductive organs. Nevertheless, the twin associations of women with nature and men with culture have a long history surfacing repeatedly in the annals of Western civilization. The metaphors they have spawned are sufficiently real and problematic that the time has come to seek new metaphors and images to represent our conceptual undergirdings.

---

[16]Although women have been and continue to be seen as a resource for men, it is not clear that the female-nature::male-culture association is the basic thinking underlying this perception and exploitation of women. There are simply too many societies in which women are exploited, sometimes brutally, in which there is no clear association of women with nature, men with culture. Traditional China is an obvious example, but there are many others, such as the Mundurucú and the Yanomamö in Brazil, the Sambia in New Guinea (and other New Guinea groups), the Azande in Africa (Easlea, 1981).

CONCLUSION

The Earth Mother and Mother Nature metaphors are deeply embedded in Euro-American discourse and thought, and will not easily be dislodged. Yet they are in many ways troublesome formulations, deploying as components of the metaphorical vehicle the notions of motherhood and femaleness, each constructed of mixed and oppositional meanings: revered and idealized on the one side, denigrated and exploited on the other, mothers and women in general have been perceived and treated by men in much the same way as the earth and nature have been. Through all of this, women's potentially different conceptualizations and metaphorizations of the human-earth-nature interrelationships have been repressed or neglected, however, admittedly, many women have simply adopted traditional male perspectives on this relationship. Another consciousness-raising effort is needed in this domain, somewhat parallel to the consciousness-raising of the the past two or three decades concerning the masculine bias in the "he/man" approach to English grammar and lexicon (Martyna, 1980). This may not be every feminist's battle to fight, but as a feminist environmentalist, I for one believe that it is time to rethink and re-conceptualize human beings' interaction with natural forces and their relationship to all the other denizens of this planet with whom we sojourn.[17]

REFERENCES

Ahlberg, B. (1988, Spring-Summer). Pesticide ads conquer nature with images. *Minnesota Public Interest Research Group Statewatch*, p. 7.

Allaby, M. (1990). *A guide to Gaia: A survey of the new science of our living earth*. New York: Dutton.

Black, M. (1962). *Models and metaphors*. Ithaca, NY: Cornell University Press.

---

[17]Roach (1991) proposed the metaphor of a neighborhood; in fact, she reported seeing a poster with the NASA whole-earth photo above a caption that reads not *Love Your Mother*, but rather *This is our neighborhood. Let's care for it.* This strikes me as a promising new line of thinking, free from androcenrism, and widely applicable or interpretable across a diverse range of cultures and perspectives. Indeed, it ties in nicely with principles of what has come to be known as the bio-regional movement, which may be characterized in this way: "People would cultivate love for a particular region and structure their style of life so as to live gently within that place" (Nash, 1989, p. 148).

Bloch, R. H. (1991). *Medieval misogyny and the invention of western romantic love*. Chicago: University of Chicago Press.

Bunyard, P., & Goldsmith, E. (Eds.). (1989). *Gaia and evolution: Proceedings of the Second Annual Camelford Conference on the Implications of the Gaia Thesis*. Camelford, Cornwall: Wadebridge Ecological Centre.

Collard, A., with Contrucci, J. (1989). *Rape of the wild: Man's violence against animals and the earth*. Bloomington: Indiana University Press.

Dyson, F. J. (1992). *From Eros to Gaia*. New York: Pantheon.

Easlea, B. (1980). *Witch hunting, magic and the new philosophy. An introduction to debates of the scientific revolution 1450-1750*. Atlantic Highlands, NJ: Humanities Press.

Easlea, B. (1981). *Science and sexual oppression. Patriarachy's confrontation with woman and nature*. London: Weidenfeld & Nicolson.

Eisler, R. (1987). *The chalice and the blade. Our history, our future*. San Francisco: Harper & Row.

Famon, W. (1994). *Science and the secrets of nature. Books of secrets in medieval and early modern culture*. Princeton, NJ: Princeton University Press.

Gaard, G. (1993). Ecofeminism and Native American cultures: Pushing the limits of cultural imperialism? In G. Gaard (Ed.), *Ecofeminism. Women, animals, nature* (pp. 295-310). Philadelphia: Temple University Press.

Garb, Y. (1990). Perspective or escape? Ecofeminist musings on contemporary earth imagery. In I. Diamond & G. Feman Orenstein (Eds.), *Reweaving the world. The emergence of ecofeminism* (pp. 264-278). San Francisco: Sierra Books.

Gimbutas, M. (1982). *The goddesses and gods of old Europe, 6500-3500 B.C.: Myths and cults*. Berkeley: University of California Press.

Gimbutas, M. (1989). *The language of the goddess: Unearthing the symbols of Western civilization*. San Francisco: Harper & Row.

Gribbin, J. R. (1990). *Hothouse earth: The greenhouse effect and Gaia*. New York: Bantam.

Griffin, S. (1978). *Woman and nature: The roaring inside her*. New York: Harper & Row.

Griffin, S. (1982). *Made from this earth*. New York: Harper & Row.

Hughes, D. (1982). Gaia: Environmental problems in chthonic perspective. *Environmental Review, 6*, 92-104.

Joseph, L. (1990). *Gaia, the growth of an idea*. New York: St. Martin's Press.

Kittay, E. F. (1987). *Metaphor: Its cognitive force and linguistic structure*. New York: Oxford University Press.

Kittay, E. F. (1988). Woman as metaphor. *Hypatia, 3*, 63-86.

Kolodny, A. (1975). *The lay of the land. Metaphor as experience and history in American life and letters.* Chapel Hill: The University of North Carolina Press.

La Chapelle, D. (1988). *Sacred land sacred sex: Rapture of the deep. Concerning deep ecology and celebrating life.* Durango, CO: Kivaki Press.

Lakoff, G., & Johnson, M. (1980). *Metaphors we live by.* Chicago: University of Chicago Press.

Li, H.-li (1993). A cross-cultural critique of ecofeminism. In G. Gaard (Ed.), *Ecofeminism. Women, animals, nature* (pp. 272-294). Philadelphia: Temple University Press.

Lovelock, J. (1979). *Gaia, a new look at life on earth.* New York: Oxford University Press.

Martyna, W. (1980). Beyond the he/man approach. *Signs, 5,* 482-493.

Merchant, C. (1980). *The death of nature. Women, ecology, and the scientific revolution.* San Francisco: Harper & Row.

Mieder, W. (1966). *Encyclopedia of world proverbs.* New York: Prentice-Hall.

Miller, A. S. (1991). *Gaia connections. An introduction to ecology, ecoethics, and economics.* Savage, MD: Rowman & Littlefield.

Murphy, P. (1988). Sex-typing the planet: Gaia imagery and the problem of subverting patriarchy. *Environmental Ethics, 10,* 155-168.

Nash, R. (1989). *The rights of nature: A history of environmental ethics.* Madison: University of Wisconsin Press.

Ortony, A. (1979). Metaphor: A multidimensional problem. In A. Ortony (Ed.), *Metaphor and thought* (pp. 1-16). New York: Cambridge University Press.

Pagels, E. (1988). *Adam, Eve, and the serpent.* New York: Vintage Books.

Richards, I. A. (1936). *The philosophy of rhetoric.* London: Oxford University Press.

Roach, C. (1991). Loving your mother: On the woman-nature relation. *Hypatia, 6,* 46-59.

Rose, E. C. (1993). The good mother. From Gaia to Gilead. In C. J. Adams (Ed.), *Ecofeminism and the sacred* (pp. 149-167). New York: Continuum.

Ruether, R. R. (Ed.). (1974). *Religion and sexism: Images of women in the Jewish and Christian traditions.* New York: Simon & Schuster.

Ruether, R. R. (1983). *Sexism and God-talk: Toward a feminist theology.* Boston: Beacon.

Sale, K. (1982). *Dwellers in the land. The bioregional vision.* San Francisco: Sierra Books.

Schneider, S. H., & Boston, P. J. (Eds.). (1991). *Scientists on Gaia.* New York: Bantam.

Schön, D. A. (1979). Generative metaphor: A perspective on problem-setting in social policy. In A. Ortony (Ed.), *Language and thought* (pp. 254-283). New York: Cambridge University Press.

Seager, J. (1993). *Earth follies. Coming to feminist terms with the global environmental crisis.* New York: Routledge.

Spretnak, C. (Ed.). (1982). *The politics of women's spirituality: Essays on the rise of spiritual power within the feminist movement.* Garden City, NY: Anchor Press.

Sweetser, E. (1990). *From etymology to pragmatics. Metaphorical and cultural aspects of semantic structure.* New York: Cambridge University Press.

Thompson, W. I. (Ed.). (1987). *Gaia, a way of knowing: Political implications of a new biology.* Great Barrington, MA: Lindisfarne Press.

Tobias, M. (1990). *Voice of the planet.* New York: Bantam.

Weigle, M. (1989). *Creation and procreation: Feminist reflections on mythologies of cosmogony and parturition.* Philadelphia: University of Pennsylvania Press.

7

HIT OR MYTH:
THE PERPETRATION OF POPULAR
JAPANESE STEREOTYPES IN
JAPAN-PUBLISHED ENGLISH
TEXTBOOKS

DEBORAH FOREMAN-TAKANO

A number of years ago while thumbing through a popular U.S. reference book of word and phrase origins, I came across the following meaning for the word banzai:

> banzai. The war cry "Banzai!" meant "May you live ten thousand years!" The Japanese, with a logic incomprehensible to Western minds, used to shout it when launching a suicide attack.

Quite apart from the fact that this explanation conveys no information as to how the word is used today (as a congratulatory

119

cheer), it inaccurately describes its original use[1] and is gratuitously insulting besides. I wrote to the publisher remarking on this, supplying the correct information, and suggesting that the author not necessarily take my word for it but look it up himself.

The second and latest edition of the book was published in 1988, with the definition unchanged.

At that point, I began to be particularly wary of those venerated books whose contents form the canon of our developing belief systems and define the parameters of our thinking. After all, we invest these books—reference books, textbooks—with a certain amount of authority, which comes from our expecting them not to be prescriptive, but to represent a valid, relatively objective treatment. With those that do not, we are not always so fortunate as to have the sort of red flag we have in the just given definition; the books abuse their authority by taking advantage of our need to use them.

In the banzai definition, the writer covered his lack of knowledge, and consequent inability to reconcile "May you live ten thousand years!" with suicide attacks, by calling up a common stereotype of Asians as being inscrutable. To someone who is familiar with the defined word, and with the Japanese, this leaps off the page as an obvious nonsequitur. But reference books and textbooks are presumably not for people already familiar with a subject. Moreover, the writers presumably know the subject well.

That last could be a dangerous, or at least inaccurate, presumption. It calls to mind the old saw about an expert being an average fellow 50 miles from home. With regard to Japan, about which people in other countries have known very little, enough errors have occurred in textbooks and reference works around the world that an organization was founded in Tokyo in 1958 to attempt to improve the situation. Affiliated with the Japanese Foreign Ministry, the International Society for Educational Information (ISEI) or *Kokusai Kyoiku Jouhou Sentaa* described its purpose in its prospectus as follows:

1. To gather and examine foreign textbooks, encyclopedias and reference books and, where necessary, to provide authors, publishers, and educators with more correct information on Japan.
2. To publish educational materials about Japan for distribution to authors, publishers, educators, libraries, schools and diplomatic establishments abroad.

---

[1]Although the expression does literally mean "10,000 years," it is a wish for long life for the emperor. Japanese World War II suicide pilots (*Kamikaze*), officially in service to him, shouted the word as a final cry of loyalty as they plunged to certain death in their suicide attacks.

3. To invite educators from foreign countries to Japan for study tours and to assist those visiting Japan, to enable them to develop a deeper understanding of the country.

An exhibition held by the organization in Tokyo in August 1994 chronicled the high points (or perhaps "low points" is more accurate) of the evolution of errors in teaching about Japan, through examples culled from 85 textbooks from 43 countries. A number of factors lent deceptive legitimacy to the depictions. Photographs, for example, were used often, but the scenes, from which the textbook reader was supposed to generalize, were not typical, and further, often invited inappropriate interpretation through their captions. Whimsical drawings used in the presentation of graphs or other forms of data, and cartoons accompanying some of the text, were caricatural and thus reinforced simplistic stereotypes. The exotic was enhanced, allowing people who felt or recognized any incongruence to shift blame from the textbook writers (who were trusted to know what they were talking about) to themselves (who had never experienced, and therefore couldn't argue with, what was being presented as quintessential Japan).

PROBLEMS IN DESCRIBING JAPAN

Describing Japan involves a number of difficult and persistent problems, even for anthropologists or Japanologists. The first is what Befu (1992) termed "a *problematique* in Rashomonesque phenomenology": The idea that one's perception of reality is a function of one's background and experience. As obvious as this may sound, Befu pointed out that:

> it is wise to note the general resistance on the part of intellectuals to be thought of as creatures of their culture. They like to think of themselves as free thinkers. They are wont to consider themselves to be above cultural constraints. But alas, scholars are as much a creature of culture [sic] as anyone else. (p. 18)

Plath and Smith (1992) drew a distinction between "trying to study Japan" and "sampl[ing] the lifestyle" or "engag[ing] it as a journalist" (p. 206), and dramatized the difference by referring to Plath's coining of the word "Jawpen:"

> *Jawpen* (Plath, 1980) . . . is a curious doppelgänger—a civilization fabricated out of Japanese parts, assembled in the U.S.A. by the flapping of American jaws and the scribbling of American pens,

designed exclusively for American consumption. . . . For more than a
decade the everyday world in the United States has been bombarded
on all sides by messages issuing from elites and interest groups who
play self-serving versions of The Japan Model as trump-cards in
domestic contests for power, influence or profit.

This is the Jawpen phenomenon. It is not some simple "image" of
Japan in the usual sense of that term—not just a cognitive error
attributable to ethnic or nationalistic bias that people will correct once
they are shown the "truth." It is a congeries of tendentious images.
Jawpen exists in a para-political arena where competitors wield
weapons consisting of factoids and massaged data and premeditated
news. Japan probably remains distant and exotic to most of our
countrymen and women. But Jawpen has become a highly charged
element within their "cultural discourse" . . . (p. 213)

Sofue (1992) wondered, referring to scholars, if there is not "a
tendency among Americans to regard any deviation from American
patterns as a deviation from the standard," an attitude he found more
implicit than explicit (p. 238).

Even with the best of intentions, however, creating in the minds
of an audience a "true" or correct image of what is being described
depends on how well ideas can be translated, not only from one
language to another but from one mindset to another. Plath and Smith
(1992) commented that "issues of responsibility, translation, and
ideology also complicate our attempts to communicate with colleagues
overseas. Discourse about Jawpen appears to vary quite a lot from one
country to the next" (p. 214). This indicates that they believe the Jawpen
concept of fabricated civilization does not apply only to those treatments
of Japan that originate in the United States.

In May 1993 Japan's ISEI prepared a booklet (ISEI, 1993)
updating by country the errors it discovered in textbooks since 1991, the
suggestions it made to correct them, and whether and how they were
corrected. It is interesting, although not surprising, to note that several
instances where the "errors" discovered by the ISEI, apparently working
with Japanese translations of the foreign material, actually represent a
cultural information gap. That is, the descriptions and explanations
written for the non-Japanese audience accurately conveyed information
about Japan in language adjusted for the acculturation of the audience.
Such material, particularly if rendered in direct Japanese translation,
does not represent a passage aimed at a Japanese audience because such
a passage would be based on different assumptions about the
readership. Nor does it necessarily represent an attempt to deceive its
intended audience, or to play fast and loose with the facts. It could,
however, appear to do so; the problem is that it is difficult to recognize

such cases unless one is familiar with both contexts and is able to see the sort of invisible limbo in which the intended meaning is floating around.

TEXTBOOKS IN JAPAN

Perhaps an organization like ISEI could come into existence because of the particularly high regard in which Japan historically holds textbooks. Terasaki (1992) pointed out that textbooks took on an "important, almost sacred" image since the modernization of Japan's educational system during the Meiji period (1868-1912). He claimed that for most Japanese, "it is difficult to think of textbooks as being merely a tool which contains all the important ingredients for education . . . textbooks have become something many children are apprehensive about because the books contain all the information they are supposed to memorize" (p. 97). Whether or not Japanese college and university students feel this way— or are conscious of feeling this way—it is nevertheless the tradition under which Japan raises and educates its children.

The teaching of English as a foreign language, although nominally carried on in junior and senior high schools in accordance with the techniques applied to other subjects, can be approached differently at the university level, the all-consuming entrance exam preparation being no longer necessary. Among the courses in English that are either required or available as electives for nonmajors is a "reading" course. Typical among the texts for these courses are slim volumes published in Japan and specifically designed for use in a 90 to 100-minute class that meets once a week as 1 of 10 or more courses being taken by a student each semester. These textbooks are prepared by university professors, usually in one of several ways. Sometimes "native speakers" of English, often themselves teaching at one or more Japanese colleges or universities, write a series of between 10 and 25 short essays about customs or daily life or bizarre occurrences in their native countries, or perhaps about their experiences in and opinions on life in Japan. These books are usually annotated by native Japanese-speaking colleagues. Other times Japanese professors of English who have lived in an English-speaking country write a series of essays in English about their experiences, and their interpretations of its culture. And sometimes Japanese or native English-speaking professors of English assemble into a text a collection of newspaper or magazine articles from well-known sources, and provide Japanese annotations. Finally Japanese professors of English choose a book written in English on a subject such as culture or literature or language and excerpt it, sometimes having it rewritten a bit for simplification, and of course also provide Japanese annotations.

All of these textbooks include a list of "comprehension questions" at the end of each essay or chapter, and perhaps also a few other exercises aimed at vocabulary building or grammar review.

Publishers bring samples of these books to the schools near the end of each calendar year (about midway through the second semester of the Japanese school year), when faculty members are being assigned the courses they will be teaching in the next year and must choose the books they intend to use. As a teacher of English in a Japanese school, I have almost never chosen one of this genre for a class text, but it was not for want of examining a great many of them. The contents often brought me up short, much as did the aforementioned definition of banzai, and often for the same reason: Leaving aside the question of how U.S./British/Western cultures were treated, those things expressed and implied about Japanese cultures revealed a surprising ignorance that seemed to belie the authors' status as teachers or academics.

For this chapter, I examined 13 of these "reading" texts looking at stereotyped Japanese images, expressed or implied. I report here from 6 of the texts material representing three popular Japanese cultural stereotypes (held by Westerners but also by many Japanese themselves) that have been addressed extensively in anthropological literature: Japanese "groupism"; the self-other dichotomy; and the related *omote-ura* situations, often referred to as formal-informal or public-private distinctions.

Each of the examples may seem to hold together in some tenuously logical way on first reading. But they reveal what appears to be a superficial knowledge of significant aspects of Japanese society. Insofar as possible, a context is provided in the examples; where a sentence or passage appears to have no context, there was none, as far as could be determined. Sudden, sweeping generalizations and stern or patronizing judgmental comments were not unusual in these texts.

DISCUSSION

In reference to the Japanese as a nation, the term *Nihon minzoku* is often used. Mannari and Befu (1991) pointed out that this term includes the concepts of *ethnicity* and *culture,* ideas not clearly present in the usual English translation for the term, *Japanese people.* Fukue (1991) addressed the Japanese concept of ie, "which is based on a lineal system of primogeniture and is expressed in the structure of the house," a "distinctive" Japanese system, and said that it "manifests several basic values or characteristics of Japanese culture . . . rank consciousness, group orientation, emphasis on harmony, and distinction between '*uchi*' and '*soto*'"[2] (p. 68). Both of these concepts suggest that foreigners (*gaijin*) in Japan are never going to be accepted by the population at large as "one of us." Within the Japanese worldview, to be Japanese is important, in contrast to "foreignness." Nevertheless, the concepts involved in "Japaneseness" and foreignness are complex, a complexity unreflected in these texts.

B22[3]
Japanese are apt to characterise themselves as shy. Is it any wonder, then, that they should feel nervous about *gaijin*?

B30b
. . . After all, *gaijin* don't look Japanese. They don't talk like Japanese. They don't think like Japanese. They don't behave like Japanese. Why should they be treated like Japanese?
   The answer is simple: it is generally agreed that discriminating against people because of their race or color is wrong. (author from the United Kingdom)

In the first example, the reason given for the *gaijin* being reacted to differently from other people is the shyness of the Japanese. In the second, the reason is "discrimination." It seems clear that in neither case is the *gaijin* in question known by the people he is complaining about; he is only identifiable by his obvious foreignness. In the second example, in addition to looking "foreign," the people mentioned are said not to talk, think, or behave in ways consistent with those around them. If that is the case, it could indeed be likely that race or color is not the main issue, even if the most obvious one, and what the author perceives as discrimination could simply be a feeling of being at a loss as to how to deal in an appropriate and inoffensive way with these people. Bachnik (1992) said that

for Japanese, appropriate personal and social behavior is identified, not as a general set of behaviors which transcends situations, but rather as a series of particular situations which generate a kaleidoscope of different behaviors *which are nonetheless ordered and agreed upon.* (p. 155)

Indeed, it is quite curious that a *gaijin* should even want to be considered part of a Japanese group.

---

[2]*Uchi* and *soto* are somewhat comparable to in-group and out-group.
[3]Quote identifiers are for author's identification if necessary.

L38
An American was astonished to learn that Japanese companies give all
their employees at the same level identical pay raises, regardless of
performance. "Why would anyone bother to work hard under those
conditions? It's unfair to treat everyone the same! No American would
bother to work hard if he didn't think he'd be rewarded for it." (two
listed authors, the first from the United States, the second from Japan)

M41
"The Japanese are a simple people . . . they do not bother their heads
about whether their work is useful or productive. Never be absent.
Never be late. Never argue with the boss. Agree with the consensus.
Keep your head down and do what you are told. That is their
philosophy." [attributed to a Japanese by the authors]

M43
[The Japanese] do seem to work extremely hard without knowing
exactly why. Their objectives seem to be either unclear or unimportant.
Unless the English see some result or benefit from their work their
inclination is to do nothing or to say "What is the bloody point?" No
only that, the English are bloody-minded whereas the Japanese are
under normal conditions docile which gives them a very definite
advantage. (two listed authors, the first from the United Kingdom, the
second from Japan)

G55
Most of all, I see the differences in the children and young people, most
of whom now seem to move through their automated and
computerized lives like zombies in sneakers, only half aware of real
life, their minds only on the "examination hell" ahead of them, and of
what I might call the "sararyman hell" beyond that for the rest of their
working lives. No wonder that to a western eye most of the young
people of Japan who visit Europe and America seem to be immature,
without personalities, and "not switched-on." (author from the United
Kingdom)

Note the stereotypes: In L38, for example, we see that in a
Japanese company at least, one can expect one's membership on the
team to result only in one's special abilities or contributions being
ignored. This is probably why, in M41 (from a different textbook), the
Japanese workers do not even bother to think about what they are
doing. In fact, in M43, they don't even know why they are there. And
the reason for this can be found in G55: they have been automatons since
their childhood!

It is unclear what the basis could be for assuming that thinking
or behaving with reference to a group automatically goes against what

one might do or want as an individual. This assumption sounds Western and probably influences the descriptions written above. Tobin (1991) said that "the Japanese value dependence, but they also value individual initiative, perseverance, and a spiritual creativity that . . . is fostered rather than compromised by interdependence with family, friends and coworkers" (p. 8).

Judgments about relations among coworkers and between workers and their superiors, also reveal a grounding in Western values and assumptions about such relationships:

L31
There are bosses [in the U.S] . . . who behave like "Oriental despots," hating to be disagreed with. They will transfer people they dislike or else pile work on them.

L63
The Japanese mentality does not find anything wrong with being lost inside a group. (two listed authors, the first from the United States, the second from Japan)

The U.S. Department of Education (1991), in its report "Japanese Education Today," stated that "To most Westerners, a high degree of behavioral conformity is typically associated with top-down control. However . . . [in Japan] instead, the cultural emphasis on harmony and hard work requires that each individual within the system be a willing contributor to the group's effort" (p. 144). It is difficult to reconcile such a description with the idea of the "Oriental despot" referred to in L31, or with the idea of being "lost," mentioned in L63.

Students using these textbooks may on occasion find themselves bludgeoned with material such as the following:

A2930
Here, then, is what democracy in England really means—heated debate, deep discussion and logical argument, carried on under certain reasonable rules and disciplines by selected representatives of the public. The sharp edges of raw power are constantly softened or tempered by the existence of balancing forces: . . . extremes of action, emotion and thought are avoided. It is this dual balance which gives England its reputation for stability, reasonableness and calmness. English democracy is a two-way process of give and take.

The element of "debate" is thus of paramount importance. This is not the same as the Japanese "consensus of opinion." . . . Decisions are made on the basis of reality, on common sense, rather than upon "that which will satisfy the most people," which often seems to be the Japanese way. (author from the United Kingdom)

Making "debate" and "consensus of opinion" antithetical concepts, as this extract does, ignores interpretations of these terms that are not necessarily contrasting or, for that matter, comparable. More striking is the astounding conclusion that debate leads to decision on "basis of reality" or "common sense," whereas the Japanese consensus of opinion system does not. In fact, one could argue that debate is aimed at creating a consensus through persuasion. If the latter, it could be said that making the decision making a public display is not necessarily better than less public, but equally fair, methods.

An example of this is the Japanese custom of *nemawashi*, a process through which all relevant people are consulted, in private, about their ideas on a matter in order to get a feeling for the needs and desires of each individual and try to provide for them in the final configuration. Group membership allows one to participate in this procedure that takes account of one's personal ideas and preferences without subjecting them to the possibility of public ridicule. Nothing here precludes ideas being considered critically, just because they may not be aired for the first time at a public meeting.

In fact, the role of the public and private selves in Japanese society is in some respects quite different from Western ideas and ideals (Tobin, 1992), making culturocentrically loaded generalities at best difficult to understand.

D41

[Americans] tend to view the Japanese [because of their keeping differences of opinion to a minimum or agreeing readily with others] as hypocrites, or else discount their opinions as not being their own, but as what they think people want to hear. This even goes for Americans who live and work in Japan. They know that agreement does not necessarily express people's actual opinions. Americans take things at their face value. This means speaking your mind frankly and honestly, to agree with what is right and to oppose what is wrong.

The cultural stereotypes both of Americans and Japanese here are so obvious they need little comment. But the levels of failure to comprehend are illustrated even better by the next excerpt, from the same authors.

D65

The Japanese view "public" and "private" as being compatible. At the very least, they feel there should be cooperation between the two. The American attitude is the opposite. They feel public and private to be in opposition, even in conflict with each other. (four listed authors, the first two from the United States, the second two from Japan)

One might well wonder, looking at D65, what it is supposed to mean, especially in light of the passage in D41. If Americans believe, as is written in D41, that it is important to "[speak] your mind frankly and honestly, to agree with what is right and to oppose what is wrong," how can they feel, as is written in D65, "public and private to be in opposition, even in conflict with each other?" And what does all this have to do with the Japanese "view[ing] 'public' and 'private' as being compatible" and being "hypocrites" at the same time?

The public and private Japanese selves exist in a number of non-Western-style dimensions. Fukue mentioned *uchi* and *soto*; Kuwayama (1992) described a different model for Japanese relationships, called "reference other." Rather than having a simple inside/outside type of division, the "reference other" model consists of four concentric circles, with the self *(jibun)* at the center, surrounded respectively by "three distinct categories of others . . . *mawari* (people around), *hito* (people at large), and *seken* (society)" (p. 122). Kuwayama described this model as in some ways preferable to the *uchi/soto* model, because the self is clear rather than ambiguous, and it is easier to perceive the relationships between the self and the various "others" involved with it.

Although Kuwayama identified several categories of "other," Lebra (1992) identified a number of "selves." Citing Shweder and LeVine's characterization of the self as "socially contextualized," she described an "interactional self" in such aspects as "presentational," concerned with face, and "empathetic," concerned with interaction with other insiders in a group or other personal relationship. She further posited the existence of an "inner self," which forms the core of one's personality, and need not be touched or affected by the outside world. Consider, then, the following extracts:

A75
Kindness to others is a personal matter and does not depend on social organizations. In Japan, "Charity" and "Volunteer" activities are often too "organized" and "formalized" to be spontaneous; they are advertised on television as such, and because they are "group" activities they attract people. It hardly ever occurs to Japanese people to help others privately or anonymously.

A7576
Now, there are two basic kinds of individualism. One of them is *selfish* individualism. . . . The other type is *creative* individualism. This second type of individualism is not promoted in Japan: to be different from others is frowned upon; those who are original or eccentric in any way are thought to be "strange" and anti-social. . . . I very much fear that the first type of individualism, however, is now extremely common in

Japan. The young have taken up this negative form of individualism as a way of rebelling against authorities, school and parents. This is largely because the second type of individualism is not well understood in Japan and not tolerated if it is. (author from the United Kingdom)

The prejudices contained here almost defy comment. The Western cultural myopia regarding Japanese motivations result in interpretations that are at best extreme overgeneralization. In light of the concepts described by Lebra (1992), the situations decried by the writer in the excerpts can hardly be considered representative of the Japanese. Similarly, the lenses created by the assumptions about Western individualism also at best cloud one's understanding of that cultural complex.

CONCLUSIONS

At the very least, it is disconcerting to find such problematic errors and misrepresentations in the relatively new textbooks on the market. One wonders what the purpose of this material must be. Obviously, it is not to impart information, either factual or objectively interpretive. It also seems inappropriate for translation because the expressions are so simplistic, culture-bound, and vague. What is also interesting is that apologists for the Western ideal of respect for the individual are so willing to lump all Japanese under a few judgmental rubrics while extolling the superiority of Western ideas, apparently with little recognition or understanding of the limitations and difficulties inherent also in Western cultural complexes.

As the study of these materials continues, and the problem areas are more clearly identified, the duty of the creators of these materials to be more responsible, both to their profession and to the multiple cultures they claim to represent, will become more evident.

It was not an anthropologist, a linguist, or a language teacher, but a physicist, Neils Bohr, who said, "It is not enough to discover how things seem to seem. We must discover how things really seem."

REFERENCES

Bachnik, J. (1992). *Kejime*: Defining a shifting self in multiple organizational modes. In N. R. Rosenberger (Ed.), *Japanese sense of self* (pp. 152-172). Cambridge: Cambridge University Press.

Befu, H. (1992). Framework of analysis. In H. Befu & J. Kreiner (Eds.), *Othernesses of Japan* (pp. 15-35). Munich: Iudicium-Verlag.

Fukue, H. (1991). The persistence of Ie in the light of Japan's modernization. In B. Finkelstein, A. E. Imamura & J. J. Tobin (Eds.), *Transcending stereotypes: Discovering Japanese culture and education* (pp. 66-73). Yarmouth: Intercultural Press.

The International Society for Education Information, Inc. (Daidan Houjin Kokusai Kyouiku Jouhou Sentaa). (1993). *Kawatte kita ka? Nihon no imeeji* [Has the image of Japan changed?]. Tokyo: Author.

Kuwayama, T. (1992). The reference other orientation. In N. R. Rosenberger (Ed.), *Japanese sense of self* (pp. 121-151). Cambridge: Cambridge University Press.

Lebra, T. S. (1992). Self in Japanese culture. In N. R. Rosenberger (Ed.), *Japanese sense of self* (pp. 105-120). Cambridge: Cambridge University Press.

Mannari, H., & Befu, H. (1991). Inside and outside. In B. Finkelstein, A. E. Imamura, & J. J. Tobin (Eds.), *Transcending stereotypes: Discovering Japanese culture and education* (pp. 32-39). Yarmouth: Intercultural Press.

Plath, D. W. (1980). Japan, Jawpen, and the attractions of an opposite. In H. Smith (Ed.), *Learning from Shogun: Japanese history and western fantasy* (pp. 20-26). Santa Barbara: Program in Asian Studies, University of California.

Plath, D. W., & Smith, R. J. (1992). How "American" are studies of modern Japan done in the United States? In H. Befu & J. Kreiner (Eds.), *Othernesses of Japan* (pp. 201-229). Munich: Iudicium-Verlag.

Sofue, T. (1992). An historical review of Japanese studies by American anthropologists: The Japanese viewpoint. In H. Befu & J. Kreiner (Eds.), *Othernesses of Japan* (pp. 231-240). Munich: Iudicium-Verlag.

Terasaki, M. (1992). The problems in Japanese education and the role of textbooks. *In Japan from a Japanese perspective* (pp. 95-99). Tokyo: International Society for Educational Information.

Tobin, J. (1991). Images of Japan and the Japanese. In B. Finkelstein, A. E. Imamura, & J. J. Tobin (Eds.), *Transcending stereotypes: Discovering Japanese culture and education* (pp. 7-8). Yarmouth: Intercultural Press.

Tobin, J. (1992). Japanese preschools and the pedagogy of selfhood. In N. R. Rosenberger (Ed.), *Japanese sense of self* (pp. 21-39). Cambridge: Cambridge University Press.

United States Department of Education. (1991). Japanese education today. In B. Finkelstein, A. E. Imamura, & J. J. Tobin (Eds.), *Transcending stereotypes: Discovering Japanese culture and education* (pp. 142-146). Yarmouth: Intercultural Press.

8

AGE, SEX, AND LINGUISTIC JUDGMENTS: POLITENESS AND "FEMININITY" IN JAPANESE*

NAOKO OGAWA

The universal politeness of women's speech has been a central issue in recent sociolinguistic inquiries. Women's politer speech has been attributed to women's lower social position (Lakoff, 1975), their status consciousness (Trudgill, 1972), and their linguistic insecurity (Brown, 1980). Ide, Hori, Kawasaki, Ikuta, and Haga (1986), on the other hand, claimed that polite speech should be explained as linguistic choices based not on the speaker's sex but on the function of the linguistic features.

In this chapter, I reexamine the relationship of sex of speaker and a range of linguistic politeness features based on an analysis of the

[1]I am greatly indebted to Dr. Janet (Shibamoto) Smith, who offered valuable suggestions and comments on drafts of this chapter. Nevertheless, all remaining errors are my responsibility.

linguistic consciousness of the Japanese speakers toward the politeness and the femininity-masculinity (F-M) of various "politeness" forms in the verbal morphology.

The investigation uses quantitative data collected from two self-report tasks given to Japanese subjects. The analysis tested two hypotheses:

1. Male and female speakers perceive politeness at least in part independently from F-M.
2. The association of politeness with femininity differs between the sexes and among different age groups.

The data not only confirmed these two hypotheses but revealed the following phenomena.

3. Age and sex are the most significant factors accounting for the degree to which politeness and femininity are seen to associate: The older the speakers are, the stronger the relationship, and male speakers associate the two more than do the female speakers.
4. Both male and female speakers' judgments of politeness form gradient continua, whereas those of femininity are clearly stratified.
5. As for the associations of politeness and sexuality with femininity and masculinity, a strong convergence in judgments of masculinity and impoliteness is observed for all speakers.

Contrary to the often asserted or (assumed femininity) politeness correlation, this study's results—which show clear differences in speaker judgments of politeness and F-M—indicate that there is, in fact, no straightforward connection between the two. Rather, my results suggest that it is rudeness and masculinity that are strongly linked in the minds of speakers of both sexes.

DATA AND ANALYSIS

Data

The self-report data were collected from 180 Japanese male (90) and female (90) speakers residing in Japan. The subjects, ranging in age from 18 to 69 years old, were further categorized into six groups of 15 each: late-teens to early 20s (traditional college age), mid- to late 20s, 30s, 40s,

50s, and 60s. Whether each subject was a speaker of a standard Japanese, "an ideal form of Japanese based on the Tokyo dialect" (Shibatani, 1990, p. 187), was not considered because, due to well-developed mass media, it can be assumed that most Japanese late-teens and adults are able to read, write, and comprehend standard Japanese.

Subjects were asked to arrange 39 sentences, which share the basic pragmatic function of signaling addresser's intent to get an addressee to do a certain task (roughly speaking, orders and requests), along a continuum from the least polite expression to the most super polite expression. Sorters then arranged the same forms into another continuum from most masculine to most feminine. The 39 sentences chosen were based on the 22 sentences used in Smith (1992). These 39 sentences do not exhaust the list of all expressions in Japanese that can be used in order to get a certain task done, they contain the most commonly used expressions. The task encoded in the sample sentences was to have someone write her or his address.

The sentences consist of three basic types: imperatives, requests, and desideratives (Smith, 1992). Respondents received the 39 sentences in random order (See Table 8.1).

Analysis

The number of the respondents who allocated each sentence into one of the 39 slots in the continuum were then counted. Mean scores were calculated by multiplying the tally and the points in each slot of the continua, resulting in a table for each age-sex group (Group A-L) as shown in Table 8.2 for politeness and Table 8.3 for femininity-masculinity. Means for each group were graphed to display the continua for F-M and politeness as shown in Figures 8.1 and 8.2.

Both figures indicate smooth alignments, indicating that the respondents were able to arrange all 39 sentences according to politeness and F-M, even though some respondents remarked about the difficulties of judging politeness and F-M without any cues as to intonation or context. The following example illustrates one such problem.

koko-ni juusho-o kaite.
a. 'Kaite' with a rising intonation:
It is a request form with high femininity.

b. 'Kaite' with a falling intonation:
It is a imperative form with less femininity.

Several disjuncture points occur in both figures: for instance, the disjuncture between Sentences 27 and 2 in Figure 8.1 and the one

Table 8.1. Thirty Nine Test Sentences.

Imperatives

1. (1)   *koko-ni juusho -o kaku -yooni.*
         here-LOC[a] address-O-write-wish
         "I expect that you write your address here."

2. (3)   *koko-ni juusho-o-kaki-nasai.*
                 Write-IMP
         "I order that you write your address here."

3. (17) *koko-ni juusho-o kaku-noda/nda.*
                 write-NOM-COP
         "It is the case that you will write your address here."

4. (18) *koko-ni juusho-o kaka-nai-ka.*
                 write-NEG-Q
         "Won't you write your address here!"

5. (21) *koko-ni juusho-o kaku-koto.*
                 write-NOM
         "It is the case that you write your address here."

6. (23) *koko-ni juusho-o kaite morai-masu.*
                 write-and receive-PL
         "[I] will receive [the favor of] your writing your address here."

7. (27) *koko-ni juusho-o kai - te.*
                 write-IMP
         "Write your address here."

8. (36)   *koko-ni juusho-o kaki-tama-e.*
                 write-AUX-IMP
         "Write your address here."

9. (37) *koko-ni juusho-o kak-e.*
                 write-IMP
         "Write (your) address here."

Requests

1. (2)   *koko-ni juusho-o kakeru?*
         be able-to-write
         "Can you write your address here?"

2. (4)   *koko-ni juusho-o kaite Morae-masu?*
                 write-and receive-be-able-PL
         "May I receive [the favor of] your writing your address?"

3. (5)   *koko-ni juusho-o kaite moraeru?*
                 write-and receive-be-able
         "Can I receive [the favor of] your writing your address?"

4. (6)   *koko-ni juusho-o kaite kure-masu?*
                 write-and give-PL
         "Would you give me [the favor of] your writing your address here?"

5. (7)   *koko-ni juusho-o kaite kureru?*
                 write-and give
         "will you give me [the favor of] your writing your address here?"

Table 8.1. Thirty Nine Test Sentences (con't.).

6. (8) *koko-ni juusho-o kaite kuda-sai.*
          write-and give-PL
          "Write your address here, please."

7. (9) *koko-ni juusho-o kaite itadaki-tai-no-desu-ga.*
          write-and receive-want- -PL-but
          "I want to (humbly) receive [the favor of] your writing your address here."

8. (10) *koko-ni juusho-o kaite kudasai-masu?*
          write-and give-PL
          "Will you do [me the favor of] writing your address here?"

9. (11) *koko-ni juusho-o kaite itadake-masu-ka.*
          write-and receive-HM-be-able-PL-Q
          "Would it be possible to receive [the favor of] your writing your address here?"

10. (14) *koko-ni juusho-o kaite kudasaru?*
          write-and give-HM
          "Would you give [me the favor of] your writing your address here?"

11. (16) *koko-ni juusho-o kaite kure.*
          write-and give-IMP
          "Give [me the favor of] your writing your address here!"

12. (19) *koko-ni juusho-o kaite mora - eru - ka-na.*
          write-and receive-be-able-Q-SFP
          "Can I receive [the favor of] your writing your address here, I wonder?"

13. (22) *koko-ni juusho-o kak -e -masu?*
          write-be-able-PL
          "Can you write your address here?"

14. (24) *koko-ni juusho-o kaite mora - e -masu -ka.*
          write-and receive-be-able-PL -Q
          "Can I receive [the favor of] your writing your address here?"

15. (26) *koko-ni juusho-o kaite kure-masu-ka.*
          write-and give-PL-Q
          "Will you give [me the favor of] your writing of your address here?"

16. (27) *koko-ni juusho-o kai - te.*
          write-IMP
          "Write your address here [,please]."

17. (29) *koko-ni juusho-o kaite itadak-eru?*
          write-and receive-be-able
          "Is it possible to receive [the favor of] your writing your address here?"

18. (30) *koko-ni juusho-o kaite itadak-e-masu?*
          write-and receive-be-able-PL
          "Will it be possible to receive [the favor of] your writing your address here?"

19. (31) *koko-ni juusho-o kaite itadak-e-masu-deshoo-ka.*
          write-and receive-be-able-PL-Q
          "Would it be possible to receive [the favor of] your writing your address here?"

Table 8.1. Thirty Nine Test Sentences (con't.).

20. (34)   *koko-ni juusho-o kaite choodai.*
                    write-and give
            "Write your address here, will you?"
21. (38)   *koko-ni juusho-o kak - eru -ka -na.*
                    write-be-able-whether-SFP
            "Can you write your address here, I wonder."
22. (39)   *koko-ni juusho-o kaite mora-eru-kashira.*
                    write-and receive-be-able-wonder
            "I wonder whether I could receive [the favor of] your writing your
            address here."

Desideratives

1. (12)   *koko-ni juusho-o kaite hoshii-desu.*
                    write-and want-PL
            "I would like you to write your address here."
2. (13)   *koko-ni juusho-o kaite hoshii.*
                    write-and want
            "I want you to write your address here."
3. (15)   *koko-ni juusho-o kaite itadak-itai.*
                    write-and receive-want
            "I want to receive [the favor of] your writing your address here."
4. (20)   *koko-ni juusho-o kaite hoshii-na.*
                    write-and want-SFP
            " I wish you could write your address here."
5. (25)   *koko-ni juusho-o kaite morai-tai-n-desu-ga.*
                    write-and receive-want- -PL-but
            "I would like to receive [the favor of] your writing your address here."
6. (28)   *koko-ni juusho-o kaite itadaki-tai-nda-kedo.*
                    write-and receive-want- -but
            "I'd kike to receive [the favor of] your writing your address here, but . . ."
7. (32)   *koko-ni juusho-o kaite hoshii-nda-kedo.*
                    write-and want- -but
            "I want you to write your address here, but . . ."
8. (33)   *koko-ni juusho-o kaite hoshii-ndesu-ga.*
                    write-and want—PL-but
            "I want you to write your address here, but . . ."
9. (35)   *koko-ni juusho-o kaite morai-tai.*
                    write-and receive-want
            I want you to write your address here."

---

aThe following abbreviations are used in the word-for-word (mostly) glosses of the
Japanese sentences.
AUX: auxiliary verb
COP: copula
HUM: humble verb ending
IMP: imperative verb ending

Table 8.1. Thirty Nine Test Sentences (con't.).

LOC:	locative case marker
NOM:	nominalizer
O:	objet case marker
PL:	polite verb ending
SFP:	sentence-final particle

Note: The numbers in ( ) are the numbers given in the task paper and are referred to in the data. Each sentence meaning roughly "(Please) write (your) address," only the direct translation of each Japanese sentence is given.

between Sentences 18 and 1 in Figure 8.2. Although the judgmental difficulty of Sentence 27 was noted previously, no significance was detected in these disjuncture points with respect to the pragmatic boundary: For example, one might speculate that the continuum up until Sentence 27 would be all imperatives and sentences from Example 2 on all requests, but this is not the case (see Fig. 8.1). As shown, a request sentence (Sentence 16) is on the less polite domain of the continuum than the disjuncture of Sentences 27 and 2.

(27) *koko-ni juusho-o kaite.* (imperative)
 (2) *koko-ni juusho-o kak-eru?* (request)
(16) *koko-ni juusho-o kaite kure.* (request)

Similarly, the disjuncture between Sentences 18 and 1 indicates no pragmatic boundary.

(18) *koko-ni juusho-o kak-anai-ka.* (imperative)
 (1) *koko-ni juusho-o kaku-yooni.* (imperative)

As might be expected, imperatives seem strongly associated with less politeness as shown in Figure 8.1 where all the imperative sentences (Sentences 1, 3, 17, 18, 21, 23, 35, 36, and 37) occur in the least/less polite areas in the continua. This confirms the claim by Martin (1975) and Ogawa et al. (1982) cited in Smith (1992) that "both requests and desideratives are considered more polite than imperative forms" (p. 64). The imperative forms also strongly associate with masculinity as shown in Figure 8.2.

In order to examine agreement in the judgments of politeness and F-M, all the groups' means were graphed according to the sort order of each judgment. Figure 8.3 shows the gradients of all group means in politeness judgment. Note that both ends of the continuum show a strong convergence in the judgments of all 12 groups in contrast to the more divergent judgments in the neither polite nor impolite zone, roughly between Sentences 38 and 25.

Table 8.2. Mean Scores of Politeness Judgments of 12 Groups.

Sentence Number	Group											
	A	B	C	D	E	F	G	H	I	J	K	L
1	7.8	7.6	6.9	7.2	8.0	7.5	7.4	9.2	6.9	7.5	7.7	8.7
2	10.6	10.9	11.1	11.6	10.1	10.9	13.7	10.7	14.7	11.5	11.4	11.1
3	8.5	7.3	7.5	7.3	8.7	7.6	5.7	6.1	5.5	8.0	6.9	6.3
4	28.3	28.3	26.1	27.7	26.3	26.5	27.1	29.1	28.9	26.5	27.4	27.3
5	22.3	22.2	21.2	20.9	21.6	19.8	21.4	19.7	23.0	20.6	21.7	22.9
6	23.3	22.5	22.0	23.3	20.7	20.7	22.8	21.5	24.7	22.5	24.2	22.0
7	16.3	17.9	16.3	17.5	15.6	14.9	18.5	15.7	20.5	17.1	18.4	17.7
8	26.3	24.5	25.2	26.7	27.5	25.9	24.6	25.6	22.2	25.7	24.9	21.9
9	37.7	37.1	38.1	37.1	37.7	37.7	36.4	37.3	37.6	37.4	35.9	37.9
10	32.6	32.9	32.1	33.1	32.0	33.9	31.7	29.5	33.5	33.6	32.7	33.5
11	37.0	36.9	36.7	36.8	37.1	36.5	37.2	37.3	36.9	37.2	36.5	36.7
12	20.6	21.9	22.3	22.6	23.2	25.7	21.4	21.1	18.8	21.1	23.0	23.0
13	14.6	14.9	13.4	14.8	17.2	15.7	13.7	16.3	13.1	15.0	15.0	15.3
14	27.3	29.1	27.9	27.8	27.5	27.5	26.9	29.5	30.4	28.3	29.3	29.7
15	26.7	22.8	25.5	23.7	29.4	28.6	23.2	24.9	21.3	24.0	23.9	22.7
16	4.6	5.6	7.0	6.2	6.9	6.2	4.7	5.3	6.9	6.1	5.3	5.9
17	2.9	3.9	2.7	2.3	2.6	1.9	3.7	3.9	2.9	2.0	2.5	2.2
18	5.7	5.1	5.7	5.6	6.7	5.1	5.5	6.9	6.5	5.8	6.2	3.9
19	20.2	19.4	21.4	19.5	20.7	17.0	22.8	22.0	20.5	20.2	17.7	17.6
20	16.1	16.7	16.1	15.7	14.7	15.2	18.3	15.3	18.3	17.3	16.4	18.4
21	6.9	6.1	5.8	6.3	6.4	6.1	6.1	7.7	4.9	5.9	5.7	6.7
22	16.1	15.9	15.0	17.1	13.3	13.8	17.9	16.1	16.7	15.9	17.5	16.5
23	16.9	14.9	16.3	15.1	15.3	17.5	16.3	16.6	11.5	15.3	16.6	15.0
24	31.3	30.6	29.9	32.5	28.7	27.9	31.1	31.7	29.9	31.4	29.6	28.7
25	32.5	31.9	31.9	31.7	30.2	30.7	31.1	32.4	31.0	31.4	31.6	30.7

Table 8.2. Mean Scores of Politeness Judgments of 12 Groups (con't).

Sentence Number	Group											
	A	B	C	D	E	F	G	H	I	J	K	L
26	26.1	25.3	26.6	27.2	22.6	22.7	25.3	27.8	25.2	26.7	23.5	24.1
27	6.7	8.9	7.1	8.1	6.0	6.8	9.5	9.1	7.9	8.7	8.2	10.1
28	30.7	31.2	32.8	30.1	30.3	33.9	30.5	28.2	30.1	30.7	32.6	34.3
29	29.9	30.7	29.9	29.6	31.5	29.3	29.3	27.5	30.7	29.4	29.6	31.0
30	34.2	34.5	33.5	33.9	34.4	35.2	33.1	31.9	35.3	34.8	34.9	33.1
31	38.9	39.0	38.9	39.0	38.9	38.9	37.9	38.6	38.9	38.7	38.3	38.5
32	19.9	22.7	21.8	20.9	20.9	22.8	20.9	20.1	20.3	19.7	21.4	23.9
33	25.4	25.2	27.8	27.1	26.2	28.2	26.5	29.1	26.6	29.9	28.3	27.8
34	13.4	15.5	14.5	15.9	14.8	19.9	15.3	16.4	15.7	15.9	16.7	18.3
35	16.9	17.1	18.2	15.7	19.1	18.0	15.1	18.4	15.1	13.7	14.8	13.5
36	5.1	3.9	4.2	4.7	8.4	6.2	4.5	5.1	4.9	4.4	5.1	5.7
37	1.2	1.4	1.5	1.2	1.5	1.3	1.2	1.3	1.2	1.4	1.8	1.5
38	11.8	12.1	12.1	10.8	11.2	10.7	14.6	12.5	14.0	12.3	11.7	11.3
39	26.5	25.6	27.1	25.5	25.9	25.1	27.1	24.7	26.9	26.5	25.1	24.9

Note. The groups are identified as follows: Group A is female college students; Group B is male college students; Group C is females in their 20s; Group D is males in their 20s; Group E is females in their 30s; Group F is males in their 30s; Group G is females in their 40s; Group H is males in their 40s; Group I is females in their 50s; Group J is males in their 50s; Group K is females in their 60s; Group L is males in their 60s.

Table 8.3. Mean Scores of F-M Judgments of 12 Groups.

Sentence Number	Group											
	A	B	C	D	E	F	G	H	I	J	K	L
1	8.1	9.5	8.5	9.5	10.0	9.5	8.0	10.9	8.9	7.4	7.5	8.9
2	21.4	20.0	17.5	20.0	22.4	16.8	23.8	20.9	22.1	17.9	20.4	18.3
3	14.2	15.5	14.9	12.7	13.7	10.4	12.9	10.7	8.3	10.9	7.5	9.7
4	29.0	30.1	30.3	27.8	29.1	28.3	31.3	27.9	29.0	27.7	28.5	30.1
5	24.1	25.0	25.1	23.9	27.7	24.6	27.4	23.1	26.4	23.3	22.4	25.9
6	26.1	25.9	24.9	24.3	26.3	23.8	27.7	25.3	27.3	26.9	24.7	25.5
7	20.3	19.8	19.9	20.5	23.0	19.5	24.6	18.1	22.1	20.0	20.9	21.1
8	20.6	19.5	20.9	21.7	19.1	19.9	19.9	19.5	17.2	20.6	19.7	20.7
9	26.7	26.4	29.7	29.3	26.1	34.3	22.1	25.9	26.7	29.9	30.1	32.9
10	33.2	34.5	35.2	33.1	34.2	33.0	31.7	33.4	34.7	34.9	33.8	33.8
11	30.7	28.0	28.3	28.6	25.3	31.5	25.5	26.9	28.8	26.3	30.5	31.1
12	19.1	21.5	21.6	20.9	18.7	18.7	20.7	21.1	19.3	21.5	20.7	21.2
13	11.7	13.1	12.4	10.9	13.6	12.6	13.9	14.2	14.1	14.1	15.0	12.1
14	35.5	36.1	34.5	34.5	33.1	32.5	35.9	36.2	35.5	34.0	33.9	31.2
15	10.8	11.4	13.9	13.4	16.8	20.2	10.1	12.9	16.6	13.4	16.3	15.1
16	2.7	3.7	3.0	3.5	3.6	4.1	4.0	3.5	4.1	4.7	4.8	4.3
17	2.9	3.5	2.7	2.5	2.7	3.3	3.3	2.8	3.1	1.9	2.3	2.1
18	4.5	4.3	4.5	5.5	5.0	4.7	5.5	5.1	3.6	6.1	5.5	4.5
19	12.5	13.5	10.7	12.6	14.7	12.5	15.4	17.7	15.9	15.4	14.8	12.0
20	18.6	17.6	10.9	17.5	13.9	12.5	22.5	20.4	17.7	16.9	15.5	13.2
21	9.2	10.7	10.9	9.1	8.5	8.5	9.4	10.5	7.8	9.5	6.6	9.3
22	23.7	23.1	24.3	24.5	24.7	21.5	26.7	24.2	24.8	24.1	25.7	23.3
23	20.3	17.8	17.7	13.7	14.2	16.0	18.6	19.3	16.3	15.6	16.3	15.5
24	27.7	26.3	24.2	24.8	23.0	25.1	26.1	24.5	26.8	24.9	25.0	25.9
25	22.1	23.6	24.6	25.7	22.3	24.5	18.7	25.5	21.7	24.0	24.6	25.5

Table 8.3. Mean Scores of F-M Judgments of 12 Groups.

Sentence Number	Group											
	A	B	C	D	E	F	G	H	I	J	K	L
26	22.3	17.9	20.0	19.6	15.5	19.2	20.3	23.5	21.2	19.3	18.6	19.3
27	21.1	17.8	16.5	10.8	19.7	13.9	20.6	13.9	16.6	14.7	14.2	14.7
28	26.7	28.3	32.5	31.6	33.4	33.3	21.8	25.8	26.0	30.1	29.3	32.0
29	33.1	33.1	35.0	35.1	35.5	32.5	33.1	33.3	34.8	33.9	33.9	31.0
30	32.7	32.7	34.9	33.8	34.5	34.3	33.9	31.9	34.2	34.5	34.6	34.9
31	33.1	31.2	32.1	33.3	28.5	37.0	28.3	31.2	32.5	33.5	34.5	35.5
32	18.0	20.0	22.4	23.8	24.8	26.3	18.0	16.3	15.7	23.1	20.7	21.9
33	21.5	20.9	20.9	23.4	22.4	24.0	21.3	20.5	24.3	25.1	26.1	23.2
34	31.2	30.5	30.1	33.8	33.5	32.0	29.5	30.9	26.7	30.9	29.1	29.6
35	10.3	10.1	10.5	10.3	10.7	10.9	8.7	11.1	13.0	10.0	10.8	11.2
36	3.1	2.2	2.3	3.5	2.9	2.9	2.3	3.6	3.7	3.5	3.5	4.3
37	2.2	2.8	3.9	2.1	2.2	2.1	3.0	2.1	2.4	2.5	3.5	3.1
38	12.1	15.7	10.8	12.5	10.1	11.0	16.1	17.0	15.6	11.3	13.2	13.1
39	36.7	36.1	37.0	36.1	34.5	32.4	37.6	38.2	34.5	36.1	35.1	33.3

Note. The groups are identified as follows: Group A is female college students; Group B is male college students; Group C is females in their 20s; Group D is males in their 20s; Group E is females in their 30s; Group F is males in their 30s; Group G is females in their 40s; Group H is males in their 40s; Group I is females in their 50s; Group J is males in their 50s; Group K is females in their 60s; Group L is males in their 60s.

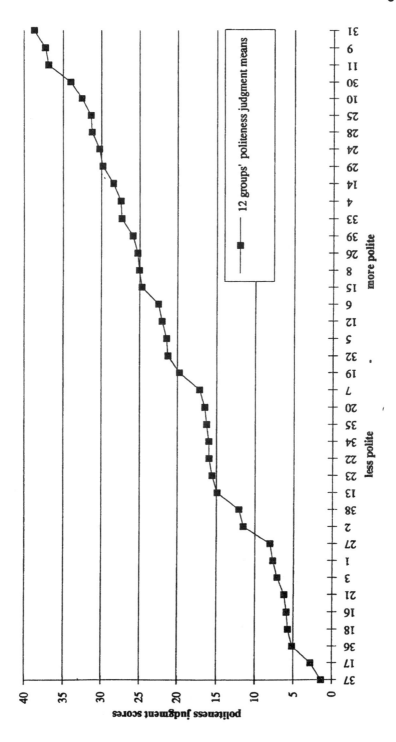

Figure 8.1. Politeness continuum

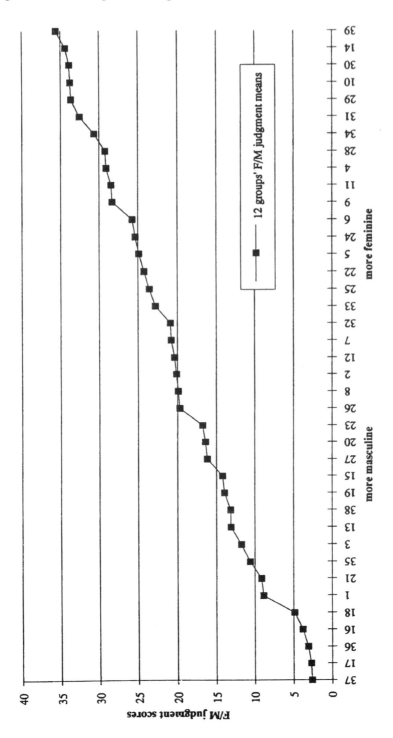

Figure 8.2. F-M continuum

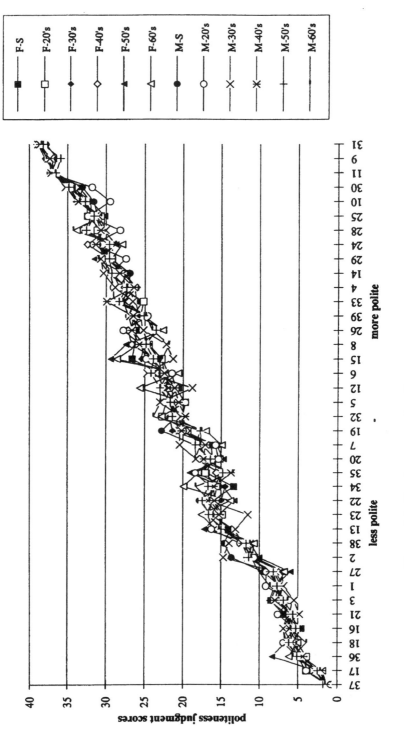

Figure 8.3. Twelve groups' politeness continuum

Figure 8.4, which shows the gradients of all group means in F-M judgment, indicates the convergence in the strong masculinity zone of the continuum between Sentences 18 and 37. Rather more divergence is in the strong femininity domain between Sentences 29 and 39.

Association of politeness with femininity was examined by assessing the deviance of F-M judgments from politeness judgments. Figure 8.5 shows the mean values of F-M judgments of all groups along the sort-order of politeness judgments.

Figure 8.6 shows the mean values of politeness judgments of all groups in the sort order of F-M judgment. Both Figures show that politeness and femininity, contrary to the well-assumed association of these two, are perceived somewhat independently.

The deviation of F-M judgments from politeness judgments among all groups shown in Figure 8.7 indicates stronger association between F-M and politeness among the older groups—those in their 50s and 60s—than the younger groups. Furthermore, the male groups show stronger correlations than the female groups in their 30s, 40s, 50s, and 60s but weaker correlations in the younger groups (students and respondents in their 20s) as seen in Table 8.3. In other words, males exhibit the extremes both in correlation with (older men) and deviation from (younger men) F-M measured against politeness.

DISCUSSION

Mentally Structured Continua of Masculinity and F-M

The smooth gradient continua of both politeness and F-M indicate that, in Japanese speakers' minds, all these expressions can be ranked according to their politeness or F-M in ways that allow speakers to accommodate to each situation of use. This is crucial, as strict conventions of appropriateness according to social situations exist in the cultural code in Japan.

Figure 8.1 shows an intermixture of the three forms—imperatives, requests, and desideratives—although an association of less/least politeness and imperatives is clear. Boundaries among imperatives, requests, and desideratives are not sharp, although there is a rather clear domain of less/least polite forms associated with imperatives. As shown by the sentence order in Table 8.1, one imperative sentence (Sentence 23) is judged more polite than request forms in Sentences 16, 27, 2, and 38.

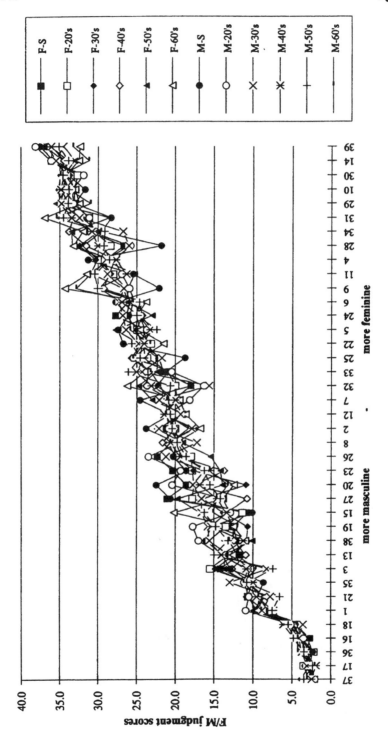

Figure 8.4. Twelve groups' F-M continuum

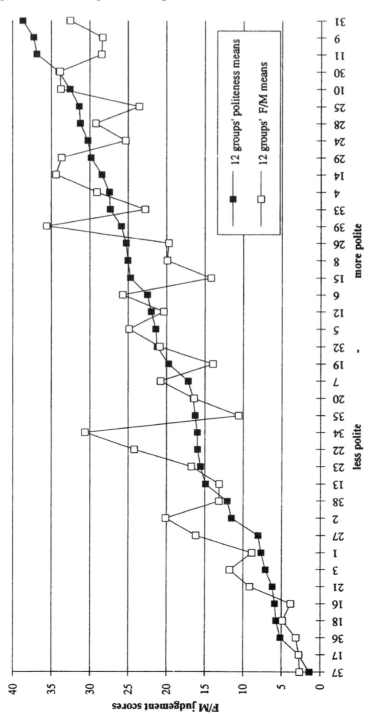

Figure 8.5. F-M judgments on politeness continuum

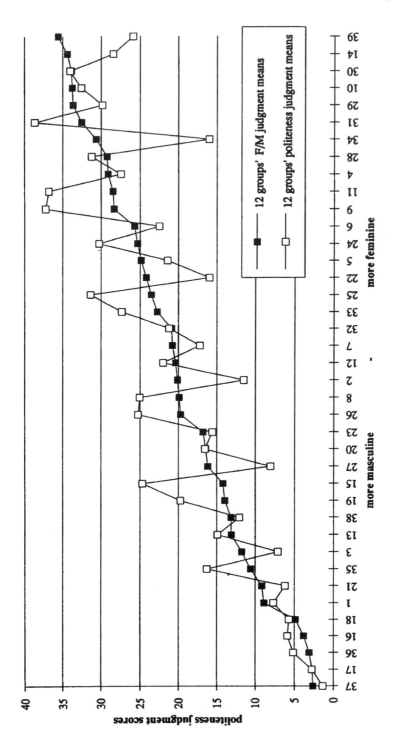

Figure 8.6. Politeness judgments on F-M continuum

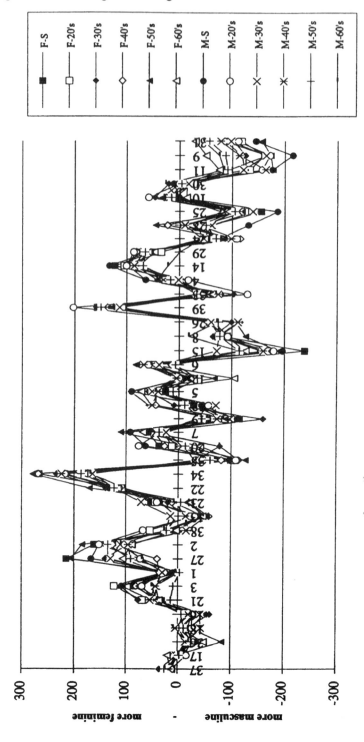

Figure 8.7. Deviations of F-M judgments from politeness judgments

(23) *koko-ni juusho-o kaite morai-masu.*
(16) *koko-ni juusho-o kaite kure.*
(27) *koko-ni juusho-o kaite.*
 (2) *koko-ni juusho-o kake-ru?*
(38) *koko-ni juusho-o kakeru-ka-na?*

Sentence 23 exhibits a conflict of pragmatic functions originating from two sources: one is lexico-morphological form *morau* which is declarative, but with a distinctly imperative semantic connotation; this conflicts with the second, the use of polite postverbal morphology (*-masu*). The latter, which is the sentential final morphology, overrides the former. Request and desiderative forms share the rest of the continuum. Note, however, that the domain of the more/most polite forms is dominated clearly by request forms, indicating that, in general, request forms express more politeness.

These findings can be applied to the general association of rudeness with masculinity and politeness with femininity, which is confirmed as in Figure 8.2. The domain of more/most masculine is dominated by imperatives with the exception of Sentence 16, a request form which is also the only nonimperative form in the domain of less/least politeness in Figure 8.1.

(16) *koko-ni juusho-o kai-te kure.*
           write-and give
           (I request that you write your address here.)
           Write me your address here.

The imperative form of *kure* is why Sentence 16 is judged impolite and within the domain of imperatives despite the presence of the request verb *kure<kureru*. The imperative overrides the supposedly greater politeness of request forms. In other words, the sentential endings determine the politeness and F-M rather than the choice of verbs.

Sharedness of Politeness Versus F-M

Strong agreement on politeness was confirmed in all age groups in both sexes. As shown in Figure 8.3, stronger agreement is indicated in the convergence of the polar regions of the politeness continuum. The rather sparse agreement in the central part of the continuum, the less polite and less impolite domain, reveals divergent judgments of politeness among the respondents about that area. We can conclude that this domain is the area where transitions in speakers' judgments are taking place. The divergences in this area indicate that politeness judgments concerning these forms are not held by all the speakers equally. Further study should explore the dynamics of this linguistic transition zone.

Impoliteness and Masculinity

Perceptual differences in the associations of politeness with F-M became clear in this study. The strong convergence of masculinity and less/least politeness was confirmed in the five least impolite sentences in the continuum of Sentences 37, 17, 36, 18, and 16.

(37) *koko-ni juusho-o kak-e.*
(17) *koko-ni juusho-o kaku-nda/noda.*
(36) *koko-ni juusho-o kaki-tamae.*
(18) *koko-ni juusho-o kak-anaika.*
(16) *koko-ni juusho-o kai-te kure.*

Four of these sentences are imperatives, with the only non-imperative sentence (Sentence 16) being a request form that takes the imperative ending form; thus it might as well be considered an imperative.

The divergent judgments of the femininity of the most polite forms (Sentences 31, 9, and 11), overturn the assumed correlation of femininity with politeness. Furthermore, the age and sex analyses show the correlation is stronger in the older groups—those in their 50s and 60s. However, this claim does not apply to the data from women in their 50s, which may be because 11 of the 15 in this age group are teachers (elementary school through college). Female speakers in this occupation, along with many other occupations such as company executives and doctors, which require authoritative behavior, need powerful speech. However, their actual speech repertoire, and the linguistic judgments they make must be considered separately at this stage. Smith (1992) claimed that "Japanese women who acquire positions of authority in nontraditional domains . . . resolve their [linguistic] conflict by empowering their own speech . . . [and] they are creating new and powerful strategies . . . on a female continuum that is distinct from the male power continuum" (p. 79). I suggest that this conflict resolution derives in part from the judgmental differences between male and female in different age groups. As shown in Figures 8.5 and 8.6, male speakers associate femininity with politeness, whereas women do not, and this is where the linguistic conflict lies. This finding corroborates the discovery of less feminine speech among young female speakers (Okamoto & Sato, 1992).

CONCLUSION

This study suggests the existence of a linguistic repertoire whose rudeness and masculinity is equally perceived by both sexes. Whereas we have tended to assume that male speakers would be cautious in their choice of polite and hyper-polite expressions because of the associations with femininity, the absence of an association between politeness and femininity in this study suggests that male speakers may, rather, enjoy a free choice of polite expressions. And, conceivably, female speakers could have uncertainty in expressing politeness or rudeness while maintaining their sexual or gender identity because they lack "ownership" of any subsegment of the continuum of order/request forms tested. Given the strong association of masculinity with the lowest range of forms along the politeness continuum men may have appropriated such forms. With a linguistic repertoire endowed with rudeness and masculinity, and politeness unassociated with femininity, male speakers can express themselves powerly. Female speakers may be intimidated by a repertoire exhibiting a less well-defined correlation of femininity with any specific subsegment of the politeness continuum in general.

Finally, the data in this chapter support a conclusion that the stereotyped notion of female speech as polite is misleading. Instead, speakers' judgments of politeness and F-M actually reflect a reality of speakers' conceptualization of men as impolite.

REFERENCES

Brown, P. (1980). How and why are women more polite: Some evidence from a Mayan community. In S. McConnell-Ginet, R. Boker, & N. Furman (Eds.), *Women and language in literature and society* (pp. 111-139). New York: Praeger.

Ide, S., Hori, M., Kawasaki, A., Ikuta, S., & Haga, H. (1986). Sex difference and politeness in Japanese. *International Journal of the Sociology of Language, 58*, 25-36.

Lakoff, R. (1975). *Language and women's place.* New York: Harper & Row.

Martin, S. E. (1975). *A reference grammar of Japanese.* Rutland, VT: Charles E. Tuttle.

Ogawa, Y., Hayashi, H., Ito, Y., Ueno, T., Kato, A., Kimura, M., Kohori, I., Koyabe, T., Saito, A., Saito, S., Saji, K., & Tamamuna, F. (Eds.). (1982). *Nihongo Kyoiku Jiten.* Tokyo: Taishukan Shoten.

Okamoto, S., & Sato, S. (1992). Less feminine speech among young Japanese females. In K. Hall, M. Bucholtz, & B. Moonwomon (Eds.),

Locating power: Proceedings of the second Berkeley Women and Language Conference held in Berkeley, California 4-5 April 1992 (pp. 478-488). Berkeley, CA: Berkeley Women and Language Group.

Shibatani, M. (1990). *The language of Japan*. Cambridge: Cambridge University Press.

Smith, J. S. (1992). Women in charge: Politeness and directives in the speech of Japanese women. *Language in Society, 21,* 59-82.

Trudgill, P. (1972). Sex, covert prestige and linguistic change in the urban British English of Norwich. *Language in Society, 1,* 179-195.

9

FEMALE-MALE INEQUALITY IN JAPANESE WRITING

YASUKO HIO

A survey conducted by the Japanese prime minister's office in November 1992 found that both women and men believe that men are more favorably treated than women in five specific areas: politics; social habits, conventions and customs; work; family; and laws and institutions[1] (*Asahi Shimbun*, 1993). The survey also found that females feel the inequality in all five areas more strongly than males, reflecting women's objections to a male-dominated society. Although by law women and men are now equal, as evidenced by the 1985 Equal Employment Opportunity law, in practice inequalities remain, as demonstrated by fewer employment opportunities for women during times of recession (Inoue & Ehara, 1991).

To explain these survey results, I first argue that stereotyping relates to the Japanese writing system, specifically the *kanji* (Japanese

[1]Politics (F-82, M-73); social habits, conventions, and customs (F-79, M-74); work (F-64, M-56); family (F-64, M-48); law and institutions (F-55, M-40).

ideograms) borrowed from China. Then I discuss how the writing system might influence the Japanese language, thus encouraging Japanese speakers to accept stereotypes without question. I consider female-male inequality in *kanji*, Japanese compounds, and idiomatic expressions.

STEREOTYPES AND WRITING

Of the five areas previously mentioned, all but social habits, conventions, and customs are concrete in that one's accomplishments or position can be seen or described objectively. Both women and men are aware from their individual experiences that society is male-dominated. The difference between women and men lies in the extent to which they feel unequal. What men may view as a great, radical concession, for women may just be a first, small step toward their equality.

In modern society, where both women and men participate in public life, they can be placed in the same category—as human beings—and so equality or inequality between the two sexes becomes visible (Ehara, 1986). Thus, the results of the survey mentioned here are understandable; women and men feel differently in the extent to which they are unequal in their participation in public activities, such as politics and jobs, in sharing the roles at home, or in enjoying legal security of social status.

Of the areas surveyed, the most subjectively experienced field is that of social habits, customs, and conventions. Carried on ideologically from generation to generation, such conventions have become a kind of unwritten law, accepted on the basis of perceived attributes of women and men. These beliefs about what women and men should be constitute "laws" such that if not conformed to would cause an individual to be viewed as abnormal and strange. The person might be derided, despised, blamed, or even punished by the general public. This unwritten law is invisible but yet difficult to neglect. In many cases, the unwritten law dictates that women are a deviation, whereas men are the norm. Actually it is sometimes startling to realize that we have adopted these stereotypical beliefs without realizing it. Taking inequality for granted, we have accepted it as the truth, and thought it to be natural.

One of the reasons for unconscious acceptance of stereotypical beliefs lies in the everyday language use. Because language shapes categorization, it plays a part in perpetuating stereotypes and in how various concepts or things are seen as different from or similar to one another. Much literature has shown that the structure of languages may reflect inequality between the two sexes (Hellinger, 1980; Thompson &

Haswell, 1977). Here, I examine some added features of the language representations found in Japanese writing. Because the Japanese language is gender-biased, both women and men often unconsciously accept stereotypical beliefs (for example that the world is designed in such a way that women and men are different, and consequently that the relationship between the two sexes cannot be equal).

BIAS IN *KANJI*

Originating in China around 5000 BC, *kanji*, an ideographic writing system, was first brought into Japan by Chinese immigrants in about 300 AD, and has since been used for the representation of the Japanese language, even after Japan developed its own writing systems—the Japanese syllabary symbols derived from *kanji* that are known as *kana* (Oono & Maruya, 1980; Sato, 1987). Both *hiragana* and *katakana* syllabaries are based roughly on simplified *kanji*, but they represent sound segments rather than ideas. *Hiragana* is used generally for any purpose in representing Japanese; *katakana* is more frequently used for foreign or borrowed words. *Hiragana* and *katakana* are hereafter referred to together as *kana*.[2]

It is not easy to tell the exact number of existing *kanji*; the number ranges from 5,000 to 50,000, depending on which character dictionary is used, but there are 9,500 characters listed in the dictionary examined for this study[3] (*Kadokawa Kanwa Chuu-jiten*,1983). Most *kanji* characters are composed of elements called radicals plus additions that result from undergoing one or more of six different processes. Two hundred fifty-one radicals were recognized in the dictionary used for this study. A radical is one *kanji* character with only one drawing that has a meaning by itself and that can also be used in making more complex characters composed of two or more radicals or one radical and other characters. Sometimes the radicals are used for their meaning and sometimes they are used for their sound. The word *kanji* may apply to a radical or to a complex construction. *Kanji* may be composed in six ways:

---

[2]The *kana* syllabaries directly reflect the phonological structure of Japanese. Each *kana* symbol represents one syllable of the Japanese language plus a symbol for the moraic nasal. Thus, for example, there is one symbol for each of the syllables ka, ki, ku, ke, ko [か、き、く、け、こ]. Children today learn to read first in *hiragana*; also, the pronunciation of Chinese *kanji* may be written alongside in *kana*.

[3]For convenience, particularly when studying characters, the Japanese Government authorized a complete list of 1,850 (1,970, with extras included) *Toyo Kanji*, or current characters with some extra, under four headings: 881 essential characters, 969 general-use characters, 28 recommended substitutions, and 92 additions for proper names.

shiji [指事] (indicating direction)
kaii [会意] (made up of meaningful parts)
shookei [象形] (copying the form)
keisei [形声] (suggesting the pronunciation)
tenchuu [転注] (representing concepts related to the original)
kashaku [仮借] (substituted for others of the same sound, e.g.,
   [燕] for [宴].

    The character for *onna* [女] (woman) represents a woman kneeling down with her hands clasped, where as *otoko* [男] (man) is interpreted as a man doing heavy labor in the field. Both *onna* [女] (woman) and *otoko* [男] (man) are characters themselves. Being also a radical, *onna* [女] (woman) can produce many other characters such as [妻] (wife), [妊] [娠] (pregnant), [婢] (maidservant), whereas *otoko* [男] (man) cannot, because it is not a radical, **otoko-hen* [*男偏] (*man-radical). Although the dictionaries list six characters that have the shape of *otoko* [男] (man), they are all composed through different processes and rendered under separate radicals: [男] (man) itself is under the radical of *ta* [田] (rice field); [勇] (brave), under *chikara* [力] (strength); [湧] (to boil), under *sanzui* [水] (water); [甥] (nephew), under *umareru* [生] (birth); [舅] (father-in-law), under *usu* [臼] (mortar); and interestingly, [嬲] (to play with) is under *onna* [女] (woman).

    But where are men listed, then? Some are found under the radical of *hito* [人] (human), which has 282 characters all together and includes 12 male-linked terms, such as *boku* [僕], *ore* [俺], and *washi* [儂] (variations of the male informal first person pronoun), *samurai* [侍] (warrior), *segare* [倅] (informal my son), *soo* [僧] (monk), and so on. It also seems, as in English, that *hito* [人] (human beings) can be exclusively males; for females, the specific representation—separate from *nin-ben* (radical of human)—was contrived, *onna-hen* [女偏] (radical of woman), to produce a lot of female-linked terms.

    On the other hand, there are 127 complex characters under the radical of *onna* [女] (woman), or 132, including reformed ones. A woman can play an important role as an element to produce many other characters, but a man cannot. Women are united as a group of characters under one single radical, but this does not hold for men. Does this suggest a woman could be a dependent garnish to make up various characters, whereas a man should be an independent master?

    On the basis of semantic distinctions, all the characters under *onna-hen* [女偏] (radical of woman) can be categorized into the following groups, (the numbers in the parentheses of each group indicate *jooyoo kannji*, or commonly used characters):

1	concerning production	3(2)
2	concerning marriage and family	7(4)
3	referring to a female	42(10)
4	referring to a male	2(1)
5	referring to infants	2(0)
6	meaning negative connotation	20(2)
7	meaning positive connotation	11(3)
8	representing feminine charm	21(0)
9	representing strength	1(0)
10	referring to a state of dependency	5(2)
11	miscellany	13(2)
	Total	127(26)

Production is the concept which integrates the three characters in group 1, [娩] (childbirth), [妊] [娠] (pregnant), which is the very distinctive feature between the two sexes that is inherent to women.

Group 2 concerning marriage and family includes [嫁] (bride), [婚] [姻] (to marry), [姓] (family name). As in English, marriage and family seem to be women's monopoly, but in English the terms are not women-centered (Graham, 1975). All the male terms but *widower* and *bride-groom* derive his counter-parts; *widow* and *bride* being the base.

The concept for Group 3, referring to a female, is the inherent feature of the radical of woman, and therefore it seems quite natural that this group has the largest number of components (e.g., [妃] (queen), [姑] (mother-in-law), [妾] (concubine), [姪] (niece), [娘] (daughter), [婆] (old lady), [嬢] (Miss), [婦] (lady), etc.).

Referring to a male, group 4 seems to be contradictive, and it is comprehensible that the group has only two characters, [婿] (son-in-law) and [姬] (husband of man's wife's sister).

Having [嬰] (baby) and [嫩] (young) as the components of Group 5, referring to infants, reminds us of a common expression of *onna-kodomo* [女子供] (a woman and her child) or *saishi* [妻子] (wife and child), who, being always distinguished from men, have been put together as one single category, and have been extinguished from the history of human beings (Nishikawa, 1987). The connotation of a woman and her child is an immature nonentity and that of a man is a mature entity.

Group 6, with negative connotation, is one of the three largest categories. It is worth noting that closer examination of Group 6 reveals that [妬] (jealousy), [姦] (adultery), and [奸] (wickedness) are all women's inherent dispositions.

To our relief, Group 7 has positive connotations such as [好] (good), [娯] (pleasure), and [嬉] (rejoice).

It may be understandable that Group 8 is the second largest category. Various types of women are described and evaluated, such as [妖] (bewitching), [妙] (exquisite), [嬌] (attractive), [婉] (graceful).

Group 9, representing strength, has [威] (authority) as the only component. Knowing that its original meaning used to be an authority in a family (i.e., mother-in-law), this character could also be classified in Group 3, which would eliminate the group of "strength" from the list.

Kanji rendered in Group 10, representing a state of dependency, have the concept of weakness or helplessness entailed from the features of Group 3, such as [委] (entrust), [孅] (weak).

This is not a complete list of the characters classified on the semantic bases, only those under the radical of woman. Sometimes a radical is used in a complex character for reasons that have nothing directly to do with the meaning of word. An example can be seen in Group 4. This happens generally with all of the radicals, not just with the radical for woman. Sometimes the radicals function to indicate only what pronunciation should be, unrelated to the meaning, as [doo] in [嬲] (to play with). Moreover, each *kanji* is polysemous, not one character with one single meaning.

And yet, due to the fact that Groups 3, 6 and 8 are large, and Groups 4 and 9 are small, and the fact that there is no **otoko-hen* [*男偏] (*radical of man), it is safe to conclude that *kanji* were originally made by Chinese men and for Chinese men. We could imagine that men made many *kanji* characters because men needed the terms to distinguish various kinds of women, to appreciate women's charms and dispositions, and to evaluate or criticize them.

For those without knowledge of how to read and write Chinese, the Chinese characters seem difficult to learn, remember, and use, primarily because there are so many and they are so complex. Chinese characters cannot account for Japanese grammar, therefore, they cannot represent well the Japanese language. Literature cannot be written with pure *kanji*. Some *kana* (syllabary that reflects the sound patterns of Japanese) is necessary to indicate the grammatical relations. From the beginning of their history, although women had little or no access to *kanji* for a long time, *kanji* have been reserved for men to work in public life.

After *kana* were invented and popularized in the seventh century, many works such as storytellings and poems were written by women. Since then, the stereotypical concept has been widespread that *kana* are for women, *kanji* are for men. This segregation, as reported by Jugaku (1987), is found in the representation of first names of common people by the Edo era (1603-1867). A woman's name was written in *kana*, unless she was of a noble family; a man's name was represented in *kanji* however poor, incapable, or sinful he might be. *Kana* has only sound without idea, whereas *kanji,* unlike alphabet or *kana,* has meaning in it, its own small universe. The woman's name in *kana* might give some impression by its sounds, but no meanings, whereas the man's name in *kanji* should give some meaning to show important abstract value. Jugaku commented that the idea of *kana* for women and *kanji* for men was reflected in the high school curriculum before World War II. Female students waited until the end of the fourth year or even later to study Chinese classics, which caused trouble for the girls who wanted to go on to higher education; the boys studied Chinese classics from the first year.

We have thus seen the inequality in *kanji* in their creation and the way they are used by and for women and men. Although today we no longer use some of the *kanji* characters, some being archaic or obsolete, we still find them in novels, poems, newspapers, and many kinds of printed materials as well as the classic books. Therefore, to conclude that *kanji* have no effect on people's stereotypical beliefs is not warranted.

INEQUALITY IN JAPANESE COMPOUNDS AND IDIOMATIC EXPRESSIONS

Vocabulary of a language is something like an index of the culture in which the language is used. The vocabulary that composes the structure of Japanese reflects the features of speech acts or mentality of the Japanese people and the institution or the order of Japanese society (Haga, 1982).

Words that seem to convey the same concept or content differ in their ways of demarcating the semantic field depending on the language. This makes the system of vocabulary coherent to the language (Haga, 1982). In general, without a concept, no word is born, even interjections and onomatopoeias. Thus, the vocabulary structure of a language can be found from the system of concepts; as well we can often discover concepts from the structure of the vocabulary. Following Tanaka (1982) , a process of abstracting from the individual, concrete concepts can show the system of concepts of Japanese people, and represent the organization of the vocabulary of Japanese. A representation of the Japanese appreciation of the norm of male domination can be seen in the terms designating women and men. How women and men are defined or represented in Japanese can be evidence for how women and men are treated in male-dominated Japan.

Assuming that in Japanese the two words *onna* (woman) and *otoko* (man) are equally paired, Nakamura (1990) paid attention to the difference

of meaning between four terms designating woman, *onn* [女], joshi [女子],
josei [女性], and *fujin* [婦人]. She also argued that all but *onna* lack sexually
abusive meaning, although the other three do not have negative
connotations associated with them. She claimed that Japanese has no
generic use of male (pro)nouns, and that the Japanese counterparts with
negative connotation are not necessarily assigned sexually abusive
meanings.

Hito [人] (human), in some contexts, is used to refer to a male
exclusively as shown previously in the uses of *kanji*, but *otoko* [男] (man)
can never refer to *onna* [女] (woman). The personal pronouns such as
kanojo [彼女] (she), *kare* [彼] (he), *kanojora*, [彼女等] (plural she) and *karera*
[彼等] (plural he) developed only since the Meiji era as the equivalents of
the third-person pronouns of most western European languages.[4] For
syntactic and pragmatic reasons, the Japanese personal pronouns are
rarely used (Hinds, 1975). The grammatical category of pronouns was in
fact developed in response to the need to translate western European
documents, and constitute a class of nouns, always in flux, used only for
this special purpose. For these reasons, the Japanese plural personal
pronouns may be the same as English pronouns (Silvera, 1990), because
kanojora [彼女等] (plural she) never includes [男] (man), but *karera*
[彼等] (plural he) could be used to refer to a mixed group.

Because the terms designating woman and man seem to be
equally paired in Japanese, as Nakamura (1990) asserted, the present
study examined the written compounds and idiomatic expressions
including either *onna* [女] (woman) or *otoko* [男] (man), or both as an
element in their written representation.

Three hundred and ninety compounds and idiomatic
expressions were selected from the dictionaries (*Dai-jirin*, 1988, and
Nelson, 1974). The structure of those was analyzed, and then categorized
according to the structural patterns. Then the examinations were made
on the concept of all the components of each category, and on the
differences in implications between the terms designating woman and
man.

The sex-linked compounds and idioms are classified according
to the formal structure and group into three patterns;

Group 1. FX : O / MX : O   sex-specific use (one sex only, not paired)
Group 2. FX : MX   parallel use (two sexes are paired)
Group 3. FMX / MFX   dual use (both sexes are included)

---

[4]In Meiji era, *kare* (he) was sometimes used to refer to a woman in novels, which
means the use of the Japanese pronoun was not fixed yet.

It appears that Group 1 is sex-specific in use and Groups 2 and 3 reflect sex-fair treatment, but a closer examination of the components of each group shows that neither Group 2 nor Group 3 is necessarily equally paired at the level of deep structure. A further analysis of the three groups leads to the conclusion that gender-biased concepts might prevail in Japanese. The following subcategorization is accompanied by an abstraction of the concepts of the components. Groups 1 and 2 include components that have nothing to do with gender issues, which are subcategorized as miscellany in Group 1-0 and 2-0. The number in the parenthesis shows the number of the components in each group examined (See Table 9.1).

The components of Group 1 are not paired; they are either female- or male-linked terms, and have no terms related to the opposite sex.

1 - O MX / FX (7) . . . Miscellany, having nothing to do with gender.

1 - 1 FX : O (47) . . . The main concepts underlying the female-linked compounds and idioms are deviation, passive, norm-oriented, seductive, bad-natured. For example, *ryoosai-kenbo* [良妻賢母] (good wife + wise mother = model for woman), and *akusai* [悪妻] (bad wife).

1 - 2 MX : O (27) . . . The main concepts underlying the male-linked compounds and idioms can be abstracted as face saving, chivalrous spirit, active, good-natured, brave. Examples are *otoko-naki* [おとこ泣き] (male + weeping = unmanly weeping), *otoko ga sutaru* [おとこが廃る] (male + abolished = lose man's face).

1 - 3 FX (>M) (>61) . . . The components of this group are derivational, and the base is status, profession, or sports that were originally or traditionally open for men. The underlying concept is that a man matches the base status or occupation and thus when it refers to men the term is not marked. When it must refer to a female it is marked. Examples: *nyonin* [女人] (female + human). The number of the components of this group has been rapidly growing. Every time a woman does something for the first time, we make a compound with female + referent; for example, *joryuukishi* [女流棋士] (woman + Japanese chess + player); *josei uchuu hikooshi* [女性宇宙飛行士] (woman + astronaut); *joshi yakyuu senshu* [女子野球選手] (woman + baseball player).

1 - 4 MX (>F) (8) . . . The components of this group are derivational, with the base being a term designating female as sex object, for example, *otoko-geisha* [おとこ芸者] (male + entertainer).

Table 9.1. Patterns of Sex-Linked Characters and Idioms.

Group 1: Sex Specific	FX	MX	Total
1-0 not gender			7
1-1 passive	47		47
1-2 face saving		27	27
1-3 new at something	61		61
1-4 ♀ as sex object		8	8
1-5 ♀ as sex object	13		13
1-6 ♀ as ♂→		7	7
Total	121	42	170

Group 2: Parallel	FX	MX	Total
2-0 plants, geology	10	10	20
2-1 not sex	63	63	126
2-2 ♀ looks ♂→ brave	15	15	30
2-3 fair pairs	13	13	26
Total	101	101	202

Group 3: Dual Use	FMX	MFX	Total
3-1 ♀ first	4		4
3-2 ♀ second		10	10
Total	4	10	14

Note. In complex characters, the order of the components is significant. The table shows the numbers used in this study, classified into three groups. In one group the sex-linked character occurs together with some other character, but there is no corresponding character that uses a sex-linked character of the opposite sex. In the second group, in each case, for every character with one sex-linked character plus another component there exists one with other sex-linked character together with that component. In the third group, the characters are composed from those for both of the sexes in addition to the other component.

The components of the next two groups are made by using the opposite sex as metaphoric reference. It is worth noting that the terms linked with female as 1-5 have negative connotations, whereas those with male as in 1-6 have a positive connotation. Even in metaphor, female can be treated negatively, while male should be treated positively.

1 - 5 FX (M) (13) . . . The components of this group are the female-linked compounds that refer to a male. The concepts underlying the components of this group are female-derogated, sex object. The female term is used in a

negative sense, for example, *onna no kusatta yoona* [おんなの腐ったような] (female + rotten = effeminate), or as a sex-object, as in *onna-dooraku* [おんな道楽] (female + hobby = woman-chaser).

1 - 6 MX (F) (7) . . . The components of this group are the male-linked compounds that refer to a female. The underlying concept is male superiority. In order to refer to a woman in a positive sense, the male term is the standard to be compared, for example, *otoko-masarino onna* [おとこ勝りの女] (male + better = spirited, strong-minded woman).

In contrast to those in Group 1, which had no opposite-sex pair, the components of group 2 are paired, in an apparently parallel treatment, as far as the formal structure is concerned. Except for 2-0, however, the further analysis of this group on the basis of the underlying concepts for subgroups contradicts the apparent fairness and shows the biased view.

2 - O FX: MX (63 pairs, 126) . . . The components of this group are equivalently paired, with no sex-specific connotation on either side, for example, *josei* [女性] (woman) / *dansei* [男性] (man); *onna oya* [おんな親] (female parent) / otoko oya [おとこ親] (male parent).

2 - 1 FX (f): MX (m) (10 pairs, 20) . . . The components of this group have nothing to do with human beings, but refer to plants, phenomena, or geographic features. They have some symbolic meaning that is stereotypically inherent to either sex, such as gentle, petite for female, and tough, grand for male. The components of this group may also be discovered in folklore or legend, such as *onna-zaka* [おんな坂] (female + slope = gentler slope) / *otoko-zaka* [おとこ坂] (male + slope = steeper slope); *me-daki* [雌滝] (female + fall = lesser fall) / *o-daki* [雄滝] (male + fall = greater fall).

2 - 2 FX (F): MX (M) (15 pairs, 30) . . . The components of this group are formally paired, but without equivalent connotation. The concepts for females are attractiveness, looks, feeble, helpless, whereas those for males are brave, capability, clumsy, independent, as in *onna-de* [おんな手] (woman + hand = feeble) / *otoko-de* [おとこ手] (man + hand = clumsy), *onna-zakari* [おんな盛り] (female + prime = most attractive age with looks) / *otoko-zakari* [おとこ盛り] (male + prime = most capable age at work).

2 - 3 FX : MY (13 pairs, 26) . . . The components of this group are taken as fair pairs; some with different characters, others with synonymous or contrastive vocabulary, which causes a slight difference in meaning and implication between the pair, such as *onna wa aikyoo* [おんなは愛嬌] (woman should be charming) / *otoko wa dokyoo* [おとこは度胸] (man should be brave).

The components of Group 3 include both female and male, referring to a mixed group. The order of the two sexes in their combination should be noticed.

3 -1 F M X (4) . . . This group is very small, but we have a few terms designating female-first, male-last in their combination. They are of Japanese origin, not Chinese. *Meoto* [めおと] (wife and husband) is the Japanese version of *kango*[5] (Chinese word) *fuufu* [夫婦] (man and wife). It may be said as in Maeda (1984) that, although Chinese word priority was prevailing in principle in male-dominated Japan, our history has seen a trend that *kango* has been somewhat Japanized in reality for everyday life. We can see the evidence for this in the fact that *danjo* [男女] (man + woman) can be represented in Japanese ways, either *onna to otoko* [女と男] (woman and man) or *otoko to onna* [男と女] (man and woman), and also that *teishu-kampaku*[亭主関白] (husband + domineering = autocratic husband) is of Chinese origin, whereas *kakaa-denka* [嬶天下] (wife + ruling power = petticoat government) is of Japanese origin.

3 - 2 M F X (10) . . . The order of the sexes in the components of this group is male-first, female-last, to which we have been so much accustomed that every time we make a new compound including both sexes, it is likely to do with this order, for example, *fubo-no-kai* [父母の会] (father + mother's association), *fuufu-bessei* [夫婦別姓] (husband + wife + separate surname). In fact, this is reflected in the title of this chapter: "Female-Male Inequality in Japanese Expressions." In the Japanese version, I used male first and female last, [日本語における男女不平等] because this sounds more natural for most Japanese readers than female-first and male-last [日本語における女男不平等]. We would not even know how to pronounce the compound, if female came first [*女男].

CONCLUSION

What this study shows about female-male inequality in Japanese seems not to be disparate from what the abundant literature on English and other languages has demonstrated. From analyzing the structure of the *kanji* characters and the various concepts underlying the Japanese compounds and idiomatic expressions, the conclusions about the

---

[5]Most *kanji* characters used for the Japanese language have two kinds of readings, *on* is with Chinese sounds, and *kun* with Japanese sounds. The words that are read with Japanese sounds are *wago* (pure Japanese word), and the word and the compound with Chinese sounds are *kango* (Chinese word). Many compounds have both.

concept structure can be generalized as follows: A woman is deviation and garnish, or a woman is treated as a sex object or in a derogatory way; a man is standard and master. The characteristic features for females are charming, feeble, and helpless; those for males are strong, brave, and independent. Because women are sinful and tempting, and men are innocent and good-natured, it is reasonable that when a man is despised, a woman is referred to; and when a woman is praised for her capability, a man is referred to. What is expected of women is to be modest and to follow the norm, but what is required for men is to champion the underdog and try best not to lose face.

If this is what the Japanese language implies, how could we remain free from accepting the concept of inequality? Every time we converse and especially when we write, this inequality underlying Japanese is repeated. Not surprising then that we often accept, without questioning, social habits, conventions, and customs that favor men.

Referring back to the results of the survey conducted by the prime minister's office, we can expect some change in the future; there may be more women politicians, and less female-male inequality in politics. At work, in homes, and in laws and institutions equality may be rising. And yet, I expect that even in the 21st century, many people will still feel inequality in social habits, conventions, and customs as is felt today unless the Japanese language is changed. Chinese priorities, however, may some time in future be represented in a Japanese way, representing the concept of female-first, male-last.[6] And because, to our fortune or shame, the number of younger people today who neither know nor use a lot of *kanji*, various compounds and abundant idiomatic expressions is increasing, the gender-biased terms may be becoming obsolete, and may be excluded from the dictionaries. It is ironic but it may be possible that Japanese people in the future will be able to do without gender-biased *kanji* and vocabulary. We hope for nonsexist Japanese in the distant future.

REFERENCES

Asahi Shimbun (1993). *Katei mo shokuba mo seiji no ba mo "otoko shakai"—ni josei no fuman: soorifu-choosa* [Women's dissatisfaction with the male-dominated society; at home, at work, as well as in politics: a survey

---

[6]We have become accustomed to the roll that has female students last preceded by male students first. These days, however, it is becoming the fashion at school for the younger teachers to make a roll mixing up female and male students in Japanese syllabary order.

conducted by the Japanese prime minister's office]. March 25 1993. Tokyo: The Asahi News Paper.

Dai-jiri. (1988). *The dictionary of modern Japanese.* Tokyo: Sanseido Press.

Ehara, Y. (1986). Seibetsu kategorii to byoodoo yookyuu [Sex-typed categories and demanding equality]. *Gendai shakaigaku 22 Byoodoo to ishitsusei, 12*(2), pp. 47-67.

Graham, A. (1975). The making of a nonsexist dictionary. In B. Thorne & N. Henley (Eds.), *Language and sex difference and dominance* (pp. 57-63). Rowley, MA: Newbury House.

Haga, Y. (1982). *Nihonjin no gengo-koodoo to goi* [Speech acts by Japanese people and the Japanese vocabulary]. In Sato (Ed.), *Nihongo no goi no tokushoku* (pp. 83-104). [The characteristics of the Japanese vocabulary]. Tokyo: Meiji-shoin.

Hellinger, M. (1980). For men must work and women must weep: Sexism in English language textbooks used in German schools. *Women's Studies International Quarterly, 4,* 267-275.

Hinds, J. (1975). The personal pronouns in Japanese. In C. C. Peng (Ed.), *Language in Japanese society* (pp. 129-157). Tokyo: University of Tokyo Press.

Inoue, T., & Ehara, Y. (Eds.). (1991). *Josei no deetaa-bukku* [Women's data book]. Tokyo: Yuuhikaku.

Jugaku, H. (1987). *Jimmei no Kanji* [*Kanji* for personal names]. In Sato (Ed.), *Kanji kooza Vol. 3* [Lectures on *kanji* Vol 3, pp. 130-158]. Tokyo: Meiji-shoin.

Kadokawa Kanwa Chuu-jiten [The Chinese-Japanese Dictionary]. (1983). Tokyo: Kadokawa Shoten.

Maeda, T. (1984). *Josei no rekishi to kotoba* [A history of women and language]. *Gengo-seikatsu, 387*(3), 23-33.

Nakamura, M. (1990). Woman's sexuality in Japanese female terms. In S. Ide & N. H. McGloin (Eds.), *Aspects of Japanese women's language* (pp. 147-163). Tokyo: Kuroshio.

Nelson, A. N. (1974). *The modern reader's Japanese-English character dictionary.* Tokyo: Charles E. Tuttle.

Nishikawa, N. (1987). *Shiro no kaiki* [Le Blanc revient]. Tokyo: Shinyoosha.

Oono, S., & Maruya, S. (Eds.). (1980). *Nihongo no sekai* [The world of Japanese]; Vol 1 - *Nihongo no seiritsu* [The Formation of Japanese], Vol 3 - *Chuugoku no kanji* [Chinese Characters in China], Vol 4 - *Nihon no kanji* [Chinese Characters in Japan], Vol 5 - *Kana* [The Japanese syllabary symbols]. Tokyo: Chuuookooronsha.

Sato, K, (Ed.). (1987). *Kanji kooza* [Lectures on *Kanji*, Vol. 1]. Tokyo: Meiji-shoin.

Silvera, J. (1990). Generic masculine words and thinking. *Women's Studies International Quarterly, 3*, 165-178.

Tanaka, A. (1982). *Nihongo no goi no koozoo* [The structure of the Japanese vocabulary]. In Sato (Ed.), *Nihongo no goi no tokushoku* [The characteristics of the Japanese vocabulary]. Tokyo: Meiji-shoin.

Thompson, F. H., & Haswell, L. (1977). Sex-role stereotyping in English usage. *Sex Roles, 3*(3), 257-263.

Part Two

SILENCED/ALTERED VOICES

10

SEXISM IN JAPANESE SOCIETY: NOT WHAT WE THINK IT IS

CHIEKO KOYAMA

"In the beginning, woman was the sun." These words of Raicho Hiratsuka for the first issue of the journal *Seito* (the Bluestockings) in 1911 are famous in Japan. Raicho, one of the leaders of Japan's women's movement in the early 20th century, published the journal for women who did not have the opportunity to read literature. She and other women writers who joined the *Seito* wanted to prove that they were free from oppression by the government, which took away women's independence (Sievers, 1983). Raicho and other prominent writers such as Akiko Yosano, a poet, and Toshiko Tamura, a novelist, believed that women had to take back the respect they used to have in Japanese myth and history.

All Japanese children learn, as they are learning to be Japanese, that woman was the sun, together with many other stories that tell of powerful and good women. Such stories are part of childhood and part of what we all share by being Japanese.

In *Kojiki*, the oldest record of Japanese myth, as described by Raicho, the most powerful sun god, called *Amaterasu-ohmikami*, was a female god. In the myth, when she became angry with her younger brother because of his violence and trouble-making, she concealed herself in a cave and covered the entrance with a heavy rock. As soon as she hid herself, the sun disappeared and all creatures were in trouble. The rest of the gods worried about her and what had happened to the world. After having failed many times to get her out of the cave, they came upon an idea to open the entrance. The gods had a drinking and dancing party in front of the cave. When *Amaterasu-ohmikami* heard the sounds she wanted to know what was going on outside. As she slowly pushed aside the big rock, *Tajikaraono-kami*, the male god of physical strength, opened the door completely and escorted her out. As soon as she came out, the sunshine returned and life was restored once again to the world.

Because this story belongs to all Japanese people, they sometimes believe that other people also have such stories of the power and goodness of women. It is sometimes quite surprising to learn that other people do not have similar stories. Japanese people are unaware that some cultures consider women evil.

Shinto, the native Japanese religion, is polytheistic. Among Shinto shrines, which have different gods rooted in Japanese mythology, many deify *Amaterasu-ohmikami*. At those shrines, both women and men bow and pray to her for their happiness and health.

In history, *Gishi-Wajin-den*, a Chinese written record, describes *Himiko*, a female ruler in Japan at the beginning of the fourth century. She governed *Yamatai-koku*, the biggest country in Japan at that time, and established an international relation with *Gi*, which was one of the three dynasties that divided China at that time. *Gi* and *Yamatai-koku* sometimes exchanged diplomats. When *Yamatai-koku* had trouble with its neighboring country, *Himiko* informed *Gi*, and *Gi* sent a diplomat to encourage her. *Himiko* as ruler, used her international relation with *Gi* to reinforce her domestic power (Ishimoda, 1971).

Before *Himiko* became a ruler, the country had male rulers for 70 to 80 years, during which time the people suffered from many wars. During *Himiko*'s rule, the wars ended, but when *Himiko* died, a man became ruler, and the wars started again. Some years later, *Himiko*'s daughter, *Toyo*, was made the ruler, and the wars ended (Tanaami, 1967).

Japanese myth and Japan's early history indicate no discrimination against women. Both myth and history show that women in ancient times had power over women and men both. All Japanese children are in some way told the stories of *Amaterasu-ohmikami* and *Himiko* of *Yamatai-koku*. So we all learn of our inheritance from powerful and good women. Japanese language has nothing comparable to the

English linguistic postulates showing sex-based gender that subordinates women to men (Hardman, 1996; introduction to this book). In the original Japanese social structure as seen in *Kojiki* and *Yamatai-koku*, women did not seem to be oppressed because of their sex. Researchers say gender roles were not clear at that time (Nakatsuta, 1990), and evidence of one sex superiority does not appear until the seventh century.

When Confucianism was introduced to Japan from China around the early fifth century, the Japanese people learned about patriarchal rule. Patriarchy was constructed on different values of gender than traditionally known in Japan. It was a good system for the male ruling class. They used it to build a hierarchical society to reinforce a superiority to women and to all people who were lower ranked. With diffusion of the patriarchal doctrine, the original matrifocal-like Japanese social structures were gradually dissolved and absorbed by the patriarchal one.

Nonetheless, women remained free to express their honest emotions in poems like those in *Manyo-shu*, the oldest book of poetry in Japan that was edited by the government around the middle of the eighth century. Many women wrote poetry.[1] One could still find a matrifocal-like society until the 11th century when the nobles were still the ruling class. Men visited their wives' houses at nights. The women inherited the houses from their mothers. Both women of the noble class and those of the common class were able to inherit family property, therefore, it was still possible for women to be financially independent (Nakatsuta, 1990). Noble women were highly educated and played an important role in the flourishing Japanese literature of the medieval era. One of the greatest novels in Japan, *Tale of Genji*, was written by *Murasaki-shikibu*, a woman who served one of queens during the very early 11th century. Such women's achievements show that the social position of women in informal society was still valued.

By the middle of the 11th century, the Samurai had established themselves as a warrior class, including some of the already existing noble families. When the warriors became the ruling class in the beginning of the 13th century, some women in the warrior class became heads of their clans. Women of the noble and warrior classes at that time still retained their family property, whereas women in the ordinary class lost much of their their power at home. The men in the ordinary classes

---

[1]One source in English is *The Thirty-six Immortal Women Poets* with illustrations by Choobunsai Eishi, with introduction, commentaries, and translations by Andrew J. Pekarik, featuring 36 immortal women poets dating from the ninth century through the mid-13th century, presented in calligraphy from 1797 by girls between the ages of 6 and 15.

were taxed to work as laborers as a portion of the tax, building important national structures such as bridges and roads. Women were exempted from this labor tax due to alleged weakness, reflecting a change in beliefs about women and men. Around the 12th century, women moved to men's houses when they married. A consolidated patriarchal social structure seems to have occurred around that time (Nakatsuta, 1990).

Over the centuries, the original power and respect that women had historically was gradually eroded until in the 16th century women in the ruling classes were used by their fathers, brothers, and other male family members as pawns for power games. For instance, when one lord wanted to have friendly relations with another lord, he forced his sister or daughter to marry the son or brother of the lord to show his loyalty and to become a member of the clan. Those women's lives were insecure because if their father or brother broke off the relationship, they would be killed for their family's treachery. Marriage for women in the warrior class often meant becoming a hostage of their families' political tactics.

Meanwhile, although women's status had declined, women in the ordinary classes in that era still enjoyed some freedom, according to Luis Frois, a Portuguese Jesuit priest who lived in Japan from 1562 until 1595. Apparently, many of the traditions from the earlier eras had been maintained away from the halls of the ruling class. He wrote that "In Europe, virginity was very important for women before being married, but in Japan, women do not put a value on virginity. Even if they lost it, it is not considered to be dishonorable for them, and they can marry without virginity" (Frois, 1994, p. 39). Frois continued that

> In Europe, a husband walks in front of his wife, but in Japan, a husband walks behind his wife. In Europe, property is shared by a couple, but in Japan a couple possess their own property. A wife sometime loans her property to her husband with high interest. In Europe, daughters are watched to stay at home, but in Japan, they go out alone wherever they want for one day or longer without their parents' permission. [I]n Japan, a woman has freedom to go wherever she wants to without her husband's permission. (pp. 48, 50)

Among Frois' observations about Japanese women is that women were proud of their high literacy, an achievement passed down by the noble women in the early 11th century who had demonstrated their rich talent in literature. Frois wrote, "[I]n Japan, upper class women think that if they can not write a beautiful letter, they will reduce their value because of it" (p. 54).

Confucianism, the old Chinese import, was used by the Tokugawa regime (1603-1868) as a moral norm for the Japanese state to reinforce the feudal social structure (Tanaami, 1967). It supported *ie-seido* (a household system) that was a patriarchal institution. Under the *ie-seido*, a household was the smallest unit in society. A house usually consisted of two or three generations: a couple at the head of household, and their children, or the oldest son, his wife, and their children. The head of household was succeeded by his son. If the head of the household did not have a son, he adopted a male as his son. Even if the male was his brother or his nephew, he was officially adopted as the son and became the legal heir to the household. If one family only had daughters, one of their husbands was adopted to become a head of the household. The head of the household was given strong powers over other family members because he was the official person to represent his family in the formal society, and he was the interface between official society and his home (Tanaami, 1967).

Samurai households gradually adopted primogeniture as the only principle of inheritance. The *ie-seido* of the Tokugawa regime oppressed women of the warrior class who were hidden inside of their houses. Their most important role was to have a son who would inherit her husband's family name and property. Although the *ie-seido* restricted the warrior class, it was flexible with the other classes: farmers, artisans, and merchants. Women in some farming areas succeeded their families as heads even if they had male siblings (Nakatsuta, 1990, p. 108). For example, as Hamano (1994) noted: "agricultural households in northern Japan kept the custom of *ane-katoku* ['elder sister inheritance' = inheritance by the eldest regardless of the sex] throughout the Edo period and it was only after the Meiji Restoration (1868) that they gave in to the pressure from the central government and adopted primogeniture (cf. Maeda, 1993). In this *ane-katoku* system, Maeda points out that divorcing the husband was easy and frequent.

The Meiji era started in 1868 when some warriors overthrew the Tokugawa regime. After its establishment abolished the previous caste system as part of changing the feudal system into a modern society, the Meiji government had a goal of building a modern society similar to that in Europe and the United States. Modernity was ideally built on an individual's freedom and equality. The government, which consisted of the former warrior class, adopted the *ie-seido* as a civil code to control the whole Japanese people extending the oppressive household system from the women of the warrior classes to all Japanese women. In a code similar to those existing in Europe and the United States, women were obligated to obey their husbands' or their fathers' opinion, and prohibited through social norms and political customs from developing an independent consciousness of themselves (Iwamoto, 1965).

The household system promoted by the Meiji government reinforced discrimination against all Japanese women more than in previous eras; it still affects women in today's Japan. Women today struggle with discrimination against them in a society that has substantially institutionalized the patriarchal system based on Confucianism and elements from the sexism of Europe and the United States.

What is the position of Japanese women today? A housewife is called *Shufu* (a master woman). Although it is, of course, not true for all Japanese households, *Shufu* has absolute responsibility within the house. Men dominated in the patriarchal formal society, but there has always been a tendency that women decide the activity within a house, part of our inheritance from the powerful and good women who founded Japan. Education for children is one of the responsibility for mothers. This tradition was promoted by Meiji government that reinforced Japanese women's activities within the home (Uno, 1993).

Shufu is often called the "minister of finance" in a family because she manages the financial affairs. A husband, except in an extraordinary case, has little idea how much money is saved, or what the working budget of the family is. If he is a salaried man, he is sometimes not free to spend the money he has earned. Because his "pocket money" is controlled by *Shufu*, he may have to ask her for a loan in advance and negotiate raises. Today, because almost all salaried men receive payment automatically deposited in their banking accounts, the status of a husband in the family has dropped. Before banks began this service, companies paid employees in cash, which a husband then gave to his wife. At that time, a husband felt very proud as the master man of his family at the moment when he would hand over the money to the *Shufu*. Now, with banking cards, *Shufu* is free to withdraw money from a bank on payday, therefore the degree of appreciation for her husband might have been reduced.

A typical urban salaried man in Japan spends most of his time on company-related activities. After work, he often goes to restaurants and pubs with his business partners or their colleagues. He goes out to play golf, baseball, or tennis with business partners or colleagues on weekends without his family. He returns home primarily for sleep and bathing. He has little time to communicate with his wife and children. His wife, even if she has an outside job, spends much of her time on family-related affairs. Because her husband returns late at night and often does not spend the weekend with his family, she does all the domestic activities by herself. As a result, she has autonomy at home and free time to spend with her friends, on educational pursuits, and on other activities of interest to her. A Japanese man ordinarily expects his wife to take care of him as if he were a child. He does little for himself at home. And, generally, a wife prefers a husband who is not concerned about her autonomy in the private home. Thus, women prefer men to be busy most of the time in the formal society.

"It's nice! A husband is healthy and stays out!!" This catch phrase in a television commercial aired in the mid-1980s became one of the most popular phrases during those years. This commercial said out loud what many women at that time considered an ideal relationship in a marriage. Nevertheless, it was surprising to have the pattern stated so openly in the mass media. Men may not be comfortable at home. Because the system comprises only the wife and the children, a man does not feel he has a place at home. Hence, a husband often prefers to go out without his family, even on weekends; and a wife can enjoy her own life without taking care of him.

Some typical models of retired salaried men have been displayed by the mass media: *Nure-ochiba-zoku* (a wet-fallen leaf) became a term for a retired husband. A wet-fallen leaf clings to an object and is not easy to shake off. Therefore, it refers to a husband who wants to stay with his wife all the time because he has nothing to do after his retirement, whereas the wife is bothered by his doing that. *Oremo-zoku* is another term for a retired man. It means "I'll tag along." Because a Japanese man's life is the company, he spends all his time with his business partners and colleagues in the *soto*, the formal society. Therefore, when a man retires, he has nothing to do to please himself. Women on the other hand, have spent time building up their own lives, finding pleasure through the community, educating themselves, and making friends. At the husband's retirement his insistence to tag along does not please the wife because going out and spending time by herself or with her friends was her private life. The wife often finds the previous way more comfortable. Those terms, *Nure-ochiba-zoku* and *Oremo-zoku* describe the situation between a wife who is independent and a husband who has lost his domain of existence in the *soto*, the formal society.

Through the media and in other ways, Japanese have encountered Western cultures. Sometimes expectations are created that do not match the reality. *Shufu*, the Japanese wife, has relative privilege within her home. In contrast was the experience of Ms. Smith, a Japanese woman married to an American for 15 years. She said with a sigh that being an American housewife was a hard job. Her husband always imposed his opinions about family affairs, family budgets, and their children's education, saying that this was his wish to participate in the family. As a result, she always had to discuss family matters with her husband. When she was aware that she could decide nothing by herself, she defined a Japanese *Shufu* as a king at home. When Japanese culture leaves men out of household affairs and so gives autonomy to women in private life, many women would rather satisfy themselves as kings at home instead of taking a hard stand as competitors with men in society.

What is the position of young Japanese women today? The traditional Japanese notions about gender relations, those that were accepted at the time of the Meiji era, are beginning to be challenged. Young people are living different patterns. Television, magazines, and cartoons show new ideal types of Japanese women. A new dating strategy for young Japanese women popularized by the mass media was to date several boyfriends for different purposes. The different roles of the boyfriends are reflected in slang terms. *Assy-kun* provides car transportation, *Messy-kun* is for dining out (he pays the bill), and *Mitugu-kun* buys clothes and accessories for her. All of these popular terms appeared in the late 1980s and seem to challenge the current perceptions about women and men.

Today's Japanese women have been subordinated in the *soto*, the formal world. The centuries of transition to patriarchy have also muted the voices of the good and powerful women of the early history of Japan. Now we are trying dissolve at least some aspects of the patriarchy. After World War II, the *ie-seido* (the household system) was abolished, and women were given the same legal rights as men. While some *Shufu*, especially in urban cities, enjoy their autonomy at their home, and some young women take a type of power over their male friends, women's privilege remains limited to the private sphere. The current Japanese social system is better for women than the one of the last few centuries, but not as good as the ancient time when women were not discriminated against in society because of their sex.

I hope that the echo of the Japanese women in history encourages Japanese women in the modern era to take back the respect for themselves that is their heritage, to create for themselves a structure that reestablishes original Japanese values that recognized women of power and goodness.

REFERENCES

Frois, L. (1994). *European culture and Japanese culture.* Tokyo: Iwanami.
Hamano, S. (1994, October). *Response to panel: Voices from the Japanese.* Presentation at the annual conference of the Organization for the Study of Communication, Language and Gender, University of Florida, Gainesville, Florida.

Hardman, M. J. (1996). The sexist circuits of English. *The Humanist, 56*(2), 25-32.

Ishimoda, S. (1971). *Ancient states in Japan*. Tokyo: Iwanami.

Iwamoto, Y. (1965). Modern power structure. In Y. Nakamura (Ed.), *Social history* (pp. 250-270). Tokyo: Yamakawa Shuppan-sha.

Maeda, T. (1993). *Onna aa ie o tuau toki* [When inheritance takes place through a woman]. Lawrence: Kansas University Press.

Nakatsuta, K. (1990). Sex in history. *Women's Studies, 1*, 98-112.

Sievers, S. (1983). *Flowers in salt*. Stanford, CA: Stanford University Press.

Tanaami, H. (1967). *New Japanese history*. Tokyo: Ohbun-sha.

Uno, K. (1993). The death of "good wife, wise mother"? In A. Gordon (Ed.), *Postwar Japan as history* (pp. 293-322). Berkeley: University of California Press.

11

THE IDENTITY OF KANNADIGAS WOMEN: A STUDY OF KINSHIP AND ADDRESSAL SYSTEMS

SUSAN K. SHEAR

Kannada is a Dravidian language spoken in southern India. Kannada is the official language of Karnataka State in India. The Kannadigas people have a unique culture that is reflected in the structure and use of their language. The Kannadigas people are mainly Hindus and Lingayats.[1] Despite the philosophical differences between Hindus and Lingayats, they share a common heritage—their language—which serves to unite them. In this chapter, I discuss the aspects of worldview that Kannadigas society shares in relation to the status of women and their

---

[1]Lingayats are followers of a 12th-century religious and social reform movement of Shivite Hindus who protest all discrimination based on caste, creed, gender, or religion.

place as active participating members in this society. The status and role of women in Kannadigas society can be perceived by examining the kinship terms and addressal systems in Kannada.

KINSHIP

Kinship in Kannadigas society is based on the principle of cross-cousin marriages; a woman ideally marries her cross cousin, her mother's brother's son or her father's sister's son. Any relation originating from a parent's opposite-sex sibling within plus or minus one generation of an individual is eligible for marriage to that individual as the relationship is considered more distant.

Marriage to parallel cousins, a mother's sister's son or a father's brother's son, is strictly forbidden, as these parallel cousins bear the same relationship to the individual as would a sister or brother. Relationships originating from a parent's same sex sibling are: (a) at generation-plus-one-equivalent to that of a parent, (b) at the same-generation-equivalent to that of a sibling, and (c) at the minus-one-generation-equivalent to that of a child.

These relationships are best illustrated as two intersecting planes—the plane of the individual and the plane of marriageable cross relations. From the perspective of the woman, she exists on a bisectional plane consisting of the matrilineal family and the patrilineal family. Each family is divided into generations. For simplicity's sake, only three generations are used in this example: the generation of the individual, the plus-one generation, and the minus-one generation. The plus-one generation of the matrilineal family consists of the mother and her sisters, marked by the term *amma* (mother). Those sisters who are elder than the individual's mother are *doDDammas*[2] (elder mothers) and those who are younger than the individual's mother are *cikkammas* (younger mothers). The plus-one generation of the patrilineal family consists of the father and his brothers, marked by the term *appa* (father). Those brothers who are elder than the individual's father are *doDDappas* (elder fathers) and those who are younger than the individual's father are *cikkappas* (younger fathers).

The generation of the individual consists of the individual, her siblings, and the children of both the mother's sister and the father's brother. From the perspective of the individual, these children are all equally related. All elder female siblings are *akkas* (older sisters), all

---

[2]Retroflex stops are represented by capital letters in this chapter.

younger female siblings are *tangis* (younger sisters), all older male siblings are *aNNas* (older brothers), and all younger male siblings are *tammas* (younger brothers).

The minus-one generation (the children of the individual and the children of the female siblings at the base generation) are *maraLus* (daughters) and *magas* (sons).

On the cross-plane of marriageable relations, there is also a matrilineal and patrilineal dichotomy with divisions based on generation. The plus-one matrilineal generation consists of the mother's brother *maava* (marriageable uncle or father-in-law), and the patrilineal generation consists of the father's sister *atte* (marriageable aunt or mother-in-law). The base generation consists of the children of both the mother's brother and the father's sister. The elder females are *attiges*, the younger females are *naadinis*, the elder males are *bhaavas*, and the younger males are *maidunas*. At the minus-one generation are the children of male siblings in the base generation of the individual on the base plane. The children of the female siblings would exist on the parallel plane as they are like daughters and sons to the individual. These children are related to the individual as *soses* (nieces or daughters-in-law) and *aLiyas* (nephews or sons-in-law).

Marriage to an individual outside the family is treated as a between cross-cousin marriage, as the terminology used to refer to the husband's family is the same as that used to refer to cross cousins. Examination of the terms used to describe these kinship relations reveals that marriage among the Kannadigas people is not the typical "giving away of the bride."

There is no Kannada set of terms equivalent to the English concept of in-laws. No terms exist in this language to differentiate a relationship by blood versus a relationship by marriage. Any individual who marries is both a a full participating member of her family and full participating member of her spouse's family. All relationships, whether they occur out of blood or marriage, are treated equally for both genders. In Kannadigas society, an individual gains additional family membership equal to that of those born into the family, but never loses status in her own family.

By examining the kinship terminology, we can also see that the vast array of relationships are classified into a set of terms that define one's role and status in the family in relation to each individual relative. These roles are defined by a pair of complementary female and male counterparts. Each role within the family has both a female and male component who are equal in status and interdependent, but unique in identity (see Table 11.1).

Table 11.1. Kinship Terms for Female and Male Counterparts.

Female Kin	Male Kin	Kinship Role
ajji	ajja	grandparent
amma/taayi	appa/tande	parent
doDDamma	doDDappa	parent's elder same sex sibling
cikkamma	cikkappa	parent's younger same sex sibling
akka	aNNa	elder sibling
tangi	tamma	younger sibling
magaLu	maga[3]	child
sose	aLiya	child's spouse or opposite sex sibling's child
naadini	maiduna	spouse's sibling or sibling's spouse
atte	maava	spouse's parent or parent's opposite sex sibling

TERMS OF ADDRESS

Kinship terms can also be used to address nonkin to demonstrate respect and level of intimacy toward another individual. The terms most commonly used are marked by the choice between feminine and masculine gender and intimate versus nonintimate forms. All kinship terms in general may be compounded with the given name of the person, whether kin or nonkin. For female addressees, the most respected and honorific term is *amma* (mother), and the term used to imply respect but in a more intimate relationship is *akka* (sister). For male addressees, the most respected and honorific term is *appa* (father), and the term used to imply respect but in a more intimate relationship is *aNNa* (brother). People who are not members of either one's family or one's social community are addressed with *amma* and *appa* as the demonstration of deference toward others is highly valued, for example *Gowramma* or *Rajappa*. Even homeless people are addressed with the dignity of the terms *amma* and *appa*. When extreme deference is called for, such as in addressing a pundit, a priest, and so on, the terms *ammavare* and *appavare* are used (a combination of mother or father plus the third-person remote distance pronoun) or these terms are suffixed to the individual's name. All kinship terms used in address are relative and the choice changes depending on the kin or nonkin's relationship to the individual, age, gender, and status.

---

[3]Both *magaLu* and *maga* are derived from the base *magu* (child), which is unmarked for gender.

When using the vocative case (style used to call someone's attention, as if a waiter: "Oh madam," "Oh sir") to address kin and nonkin, the term *een(u)* is prefixed to the choice of kinship term or to the honorific vocative pronoun *ri:*.[4] Also, when addressing an intimate friend or relative in the vocative certain terms of affection are used (*eenuu-swamii, eenuu-andami*).

People also address each other by their given name or the *devarahesaru* (the god name). The components of a name are as follows: the family village, the occupation or caste name, and the given name, and in more recent times the caste or occupation name has been replaced by the father's given name.[5] When addressing someone by her *devarahesau*, the name is marked either for kinship, a vocative suffix, or an honorific suffix. The kinship markers that are added to the individual's given name reflect either the kinship relationship between the speaker and the addressee or in the case of nonkin, reflect the age and level of intimacy being expressed by the speaker. For nonkin, the term *amma* or *avva* and *appa* or *ayya* (mother and father, respectively) are used to express that the addressee is either older or in some other manner a respected mentor for the speaker. The terms *akka* and *aNNa* (elder sister and elder brother), are used to express similar age, status, and a level of intimacy. For kinfolk, all address terms may be used to mark a name, but often the parallel kinship terms referring to relationships of mother, father, sister, and brother (where sister and brother are subdivided into elder and younger) are much more common in address, than address by name. The selection of term is based on generation and relative age between the interlocutors. The vocative case can be added to this complex of name and kinship marker by the addition of length to the final vowel or use of the clitic pronoun *ri:*.

The use of names in address between spouses is rare. The spouse's name holds a very special status. Wives and husbands refer to each other only with pronouns, kinship terms, or certain special hypocoristics (nicknames). The importance of the spouse's name can be seen in the game *hesaru hel ri:* (What do you call your spouse?). This game is a part of the postwedding ceremonies and encourages the family members, but mainly the new bride and groom, to verbally acknowledge their spouse by name or to create an inventive riddle that describes the bride or the groom. The other common method for addressing a spouse is to use hypocoristics that demonstrate both respect and intimacy, such as *savkara/i, yajamani/a, andami/a,* and so on.

---

[4] The reference is to a form that is neither a suffix nor a separate word, but something in between.

[5] The use of the father's given name is a practice adopted from Indo-European culture.

Married women in Karnataka do not lose their name; they continue to be addressed by their given name with the possible addition of *srimati*,[6] an honorific marker of marriage. As a woman, she would be optionally marked as *kumari* before marriage, so the marker, *srimati*, signifies the promotion to adulthood and being a fully active member of the community. Men also undergo the same process of status change, from *kumara* to *sri*. Both individuals undergo the same process of change in status, but with unique terms that reflect similar yet different roles in society.[7]

It is now becoming popular in urban areas to follow the Western paradigm of reference toward marriage by identifying a married woman by her husband's given name plus the marriage title *srimati*, thus erasing the woman's unique identity and marking her as her husband's property. This custom is not widely practiced and would not be acceptable in traditional rural cultures, but it is growing in popularity and poses a threat to the status and identity of women in the culture. A person who is referred to in this manner is without identity and therefore is treated as an object rather than a sentient being. Adoption of the English terms *aunty* and *uncle* also lead to a reduction in the unique identity of kin.

By examining the system of kinship and address in Kannada, we can establish to a certain extent the role of women in this society. Women and men are identified by different terms in kinship and address, but for every role or relationship there are two equal status terms used to describe it, one for women and one for men. The most polite and honored forms of address do not differentiate gender; they are either neuter or plural. Women in this culture enjoy a status equal to men as they function in similar family and societal roles. Women are given unique identity from men, but yet maintain the same status as men. With the Western influences throughout India, the status of women in society is in jeopardy as with the loss of unique identity in kinship and address leads to a loss of status.

Two major problems related to Westernization are dowry murders and the *satya* ritual.[8] North American media have publicized

---

[6]*Srimati* and *sri* are borrowed from Indo-European, where the feminine is derived from the masculine. Note that the Dravidian root *kumar* does not derive the form for one gender from the other; both feminine and masculine are equally marked.

[7]Marriage in this culture is perceived as a marriage between two families and the individual members of those families, but they do not become one. Thus, there is no loss of identity nor status for either spouse.

[8]*Satya* is the ritual by which widows may commit suicide by leaping into the funeral pyres of their husband.

these problems and, indeed, they are problems. Some different information, however, might place the problems in perspective. Statistics reported by the radio program, *Passages to India*, provide the basis for comparisons. The per capita incidence of wife murder in India is approximately one twelfth that of the United States; and a woman in the United States is 600 times more likely to be murdered by her husband than in India. But, of course, any murder is a tragedy, so the root of the problem should be found.

Dowry (paying a bride price) was a concept introduced into India with English colonial rule. Due it its Indo-European heritage, the concept was more easily adopted in northern India, than in southern India. Dowry was most likely implemented in Southern India in response to the laws of land ownership set by colonial governments (Shivacharya, 1991). Women lost their rights of land ownership, so the only means to pass on assets to a daughter was to use the term *dowry* and to sign the land into the husband's name. With the passage of time, the practice became a tradition and the original intent became corrupted. This loss of female rights to land probably also is the original motivation for women to jump into the funeral pyres of their husband. They had no land, no status; many in such a situation became desperately suicidal and the funeral pyre offered a way out. With these perspectives on the problems of dowry murder and the *satya* ritual, with the root now exposed, there is need to work at kannadizing society to solve the identity problems caused by westernization.

CONCLUSION

Examining the Kannada language shows that women in the culture play roles that are sometimes common to their male counterparts in the kinship system, but with a unique, separate identity. Women also hold a status that might be thought of as equal if one were to think of it within the U.S. system of hierarchical thinking. Within the Kannada system of thinking, the status would more accurately be described as a unique, unranked comparison. Kannadigas women bear their own name, gain whole acceptance into an additional family at marriage, without losing their own family, and receive status and identity by the unique relationship they bear to other kin and nonkin. To understand such a system, we must be careful not to view it through the perspective of the very different way of thinking reflected in English.

REFERENCES

Shivacharya, S. (1991). *Marriage and family*. Sirigere, India: Sri Taralabalu
    Jagadguru Brihanmath.

12

WHO SPEAKS FOR NORTH AFRICAN WOMEN IN FRANCE?

PATRICIA GEESEY

North African women in France are currently at the center of a complex debate on the nature of integration into French society for France's estimated 4.6 million immigrants.[1] Of this 4.6 million, the majority profess the Muslim faith and come from the former French spheres of influence in North and west Africa.

Much of the debate in French society concerning immigration focuses on the role of Islam in a secular society, Islam and human rights, the future of the French national identity in a multicultural society, and

---

[1]In France, the terms *immigrants* and *foreigners* are used in slightly different ways, owing to the complexity of the French nationality code. Counted among the 4.6 million immigrants are also approximately 1.4 million who have already received French nationality. At present, French law stipulates that children born to permanent legal alien parents do not receive automatic citizenship (available virtually on request) at the age of 18 years, but they are counted as "immigrants" until that time. For further information on immigration in France consult Bernard's (1993) *L' immigration.*

the perceived "cultural differences" between the French (*les Français de souche*) and immigrants from north and west Africa. A careful examination of the sociological and political discourse on the presence of north African, or *Maghrebian* women (the term most commonly employed in France to refer to those people originating from either Algeria, Morocco, or Tunisia), reveals two recurring tendencies as to how Arab-Muslim women in France are perceived: They are either the potential agents of a smooth integration into French society or the innocent victims of Islamic fundamentalist agendas. Increasingly, Maghrebian women in France are beginning to speak for themselves, instead of being used to symbolize or support some political view. The purpose of this chapter is to discuss two such separate forums. The first, *Le Voile du Silence* (The Veil of Silence, 1990); is the exposé-style autobiography of the Algerian-Kabyle singer and entertainer who uses the name Djura. The second, *L'Honneur et l'amertume: Le destin ordinaire d'une femme Kabyle* (Honor and Bitterness: The Normal Fate of a Kabyle Woman, 1993), by the Franco-Algerian anthropologist Nedjma Plantade, is a transcription of the oral autobiography of Louisa Azzizen, an Algerian-Kabyle immigrant living in France since 1960.

The Kabyles belong to the Berber ethnic group, identifying their origins as being in the Kabylia mountain range of northern Algeria. Although Islamized, the Kabyles are recognized for their strict sense of family honor, their identification with their clans, and their strong sense of belonging to a culture whose traditions and legends pre-date the coming of ethnic Arab groups to north Africa. The Kabyles have long been one of the most well represented groups in north African immigration to France. Before 1974, Maghrebian immigration to France consisted mainly of men who worked in French factories and mines for most of the year, and spent no more than 3 to 5 weeks a year with their families in north Africa. Before the 1970s, family immigration was relatively rare. As Plantade's (1993) consultant Louisa Azzizen explained, it was something of a taboo to take women to France because it was feared they would somehow become tainted and begin to adopt French customs. Algerian women immigrants had to be especially careful not to be seen in public in France by other immigrants from their regions, as word would inevitably get back to the family that "Madame So and So" was going out in public and bringing dishonor to her family.

After 1974, however, family immigration to France became feasible and even desirable as the French government instituted family regroupment programs that allowed workers to bring their wives and children to France. All children of legal immigrants have been entitled to family allowances and free education in the public schools. The shift from guest worker to family resettlement immigration resulted in a need to address the nature of integration into French society. The issues associated with integration and assimilation gained widespread attention during the 1980s with the coming of age of the *Beur* Generation. *Beur* is a Parisian slang word for Arab and the term has been used by second-generation north African youth of immigrant families to refer to themselves, using it to suggest a sense of cultural and ethnic identity that is neither entirely French nor Maghrebian.

The decade of the 1980s also saw the development of an interest in Islam in France and in the status of women in Arab-Islamic societies. This interest arose in academic as well as popular circles, largely due to several incidents in France during the late 1980s: the reaction of the Muslim community in France to the publication of Salman Rushdie's *Satanic Verses*; the "Scarf Affair" in autumn 1989; and recurring, sensationalized reports of "honor killings" and forced marriages among Maghrebian families in France. Begag and Chaouite (1990), two Maghrebian social scientists who studied north African immigration and integration, noted that the "Scarf Affair" in particular polarized French society around the issue of women's rights in Islam and the role that the French government, and French society in general, should play in intervening into the lives of north African immigrants and their families.

The "Scarf Affair" began in the Paris suburb of Creil when three girls from north African families were suspended from their junior high school for refusing to remove their head coverings inside the school buildings. The families involved and the girls' supporters in the French press felt that the modest apparel was not so much a religious symbol as a traditional cultural practice, and that the scarves would have to be tolerated so that the families would continue to permit their daughters to attend a co-ed school. Supporters of the school policy against the scarves felt the families were oppressing their daughters and that the scarves were an attempt to proselytize Islam. This, they believed, violated the strict code of secularism for French public schools. The government intervened after public opinion divided into two camps; it was decided that the girls' attendance in school was ultimately what mattered the most and they were allowed to wear their scarves in class.

The debate about the scarves touched a sensitive nerve in French society, generating a renewed interest in women's status in Arab-Islamic societies. In the popular imagination, fed by sensational newspaper accounts of women's conditions in Muslim countries, Arab immigrant traditions in France became synonymous with reactionary cultural practices. *Francoscopie*, Mermet's (1992) annual compilation of French opinion polls, reported that a significant majority of French nationals interviewed felt that the current characteristics of immigration to France, that is, immigrants from north and west Africa, represented a distinct threat to French cultural identity. Seventy-six percent of the respondents felt there were "too many Arabs" in France. Seventy-six percent of those interviewed also said the Islamic faith does not respect the rights of women. Media attention to issues related to north African women in France has no doubt contributed to the popularization of questions concerning women's status under Islam.

Needless to say, as the media devoted attention to the question of Arab-Muslim women in France, so did members of the intellectual and academic community. From the latter group, an attempt has been made to address the matter in an objective and balanced tone. Individuals such as Etienne (1991), a professor and researcher of political science, Naïr (1992), also a political scientist, and Abdelkrim-Chikh (1991), a sociologist, have suggested that the often "paternalistic" interest of French society regarding Arab women's status has its roots in the colonial past, when the need to "modernize" Arab societies and "improve" the lot of women—victims of their own cultural practices— was used to justify colonial practice.

Abdelkrim-Chikh (1991) observed that north African women immigrants, as well as second-generation north African women in France are considered signs of a "double alterity," woman and Other, who may be doubly dominated because she is both "foreign" and female. North African women in France in her view, are "caught in the signs of another system of cultural references. . . . The question is to investigate the results of the encounter with a double alterity (a foreign woman) in a society that has erected secularism as its totem by way of the asexual individual, free, brother, and equal unto himself!" (p. 236). The notion of double otherness of north African women living in a secular, egalitarian French society forms the basis for much of the discourse involving the oppression of Arab-Muslim women and their potential "liberation" brought about by contact with the ideals of French society.

Interest in the conditions under which Maghrebian women immigrants live exists in popular as well as academic circles. The otherness attributed to them within the host society is often manifested by outward signs, the most recognizable of which are illiteracy; traditional dress including *djellabas,* scarves, and even face veils; high birthrates and poverty; and physical seclusion. The perception in French society is that north African women immigrants live on the margins of society even more than male immigrants or the second-generation offspring of immigrant families. And yet, their very presence appears to have sparked a flurry of print and visual documentation regarding the conditions in which they live. In many ways, intellectual and popular circles in France have blossomed into what Spivak (1980) has referred to as "postcolonial garden where the marginal can speak and be spoken, even spoken for" (p. 221). Spivak (1988) identified women from the developing world as being "doubly erased" (p. 287). Women are even further in the shadows than their male counterparts because they are more likely to suffer from what she described as an insidious, "benevolent First-World appropriation and reinscription of the Third World as an Other . . ." (p. 289).

The questions I raise, however, are as follow: "Who speaks for north African women?" "To whom and for what reasons?" Addressing the questions raised by each of the testimonial-style narratives by Djura and Azzizen (Nedjma Plantade) enters the debate on whether north African women in France are being victimized by a neo-colonialist tendency toward objectification and appropriation.

More complex is the question of whether certain north African women in France are consciously or unconsciously attempting to color or even exploit French society's perception of women's status in the Maghrebian community. My reading of Djura's *Voile du silence* leads me to conclude that, however sincere her original motives were in writing this story of her life, the manner in which the work is narrated, and her emphasis on emotionally charged issues regarding north African women's status in France without attending to cultural contexts, can cause this particular work to be read as an affirmation of many negative stereotypes about Kabyle-Algerian culture that pre-exist in the popular imagination of many French readers.

Mohanty (1991) noted the danger for feminists—from both the West and from the developing world—of creating a monolithic, discursive "Third World Woman" merely defined in terms of her victimization and oppression (p. 57). A desire to focus attention on the injustices suffered by women all over the world must be tempered with an awareness of the existing cultural, religious, class, and geographic specificities that affect women's lives. Lazreg (1988) reminded us of the tendency of feminists—both Middle Eastern and Western—to unconsciously "speak for" the very women whose subjectivity they hope to restore: "[Women from the Arab-Muslim world] appear on the feminist stage as representatives of the millions of women in their own societies. To what extent they do violence to the women they claim authority to write and speak about is a question that is seldom raised" (p. 89).

Djura (1990) prefaced her autobiography with the declaration that the terrible series of events through which she has lived are nothing unusual for women from similar backgrounds. She explained that her choice of title (*Veil of Silence*) symbolizes her desire to "lift the curtain of silence" that hides north African women and renders them speechless, ultimately denying their very existence. Djura's autobiography has sold more than 500,000 copies and has also been published in the inexpensive "Livre de Poche" series. Her writing style is accessible to readers from all backgrounds. She begins her tale with a description of the attack she and her French companion suffered in the summer of 1987. (Djura has since married Hervé Lacroix, her producer and manager.) At that time, Djura was 7 months pregnant with her first child. She and Hervé were beaten by her brother and a niece. Hervé was shot and the assailants ran away. During Djura's and Hervé's recovery, she decided to write her life story to expose what she called the "absurd and medieval conditions" under which Maghrebian women must live, even those born and raised in France (p. 14).

Djura's (1990) story is one of a woman who even quite young sought to rebel against oppressive customs and restraints placed on girls who must always be conscious of their duties to remain obedient, secluded, and pure. To do otherwise would entail corporal punishment or even death at the hands of an enraged father or brother. Djura described her youth as a terrible period. The family lived in one miserable housing project after another. Her alcoholic father subjected her mother, sisters, and herself to brutal beatings. Her brothers became high school dropouts and juvenile delinquents. Only Djura herself had a goal in life: to attend a *lycée* specializing in theater arts and to someday work in the field of cinema production. This caused a scandal in the family. After her return to Algeria in the early 1970s to film a documentary about the plight of Franco-Algerian guest workers, Djura was imprisoned by her brothers (with the entire family's approval) in order to break her spirit and in an attempt to force her agreement to an arranged marriage. She writes that her entire family believed the treatment justified because they suspected her of having a romantic liaison with a Frenchman. Before her imprisonment in Algiers, Djura made a return visit to her family's village in the Djurdjura mountains of Kabylia.

Djura described the awakening of her feminist consciousness at this time and her desire to help liberate north African women from the bondage of male authority, poverty, and ignorance she identified as being their daily lot. Djura wrote that she organized women's meetings to transmit her message of the better life awaiting women who refuse to continue to submit to tradition. Djura recounted stories of honor killings of suspected nonvirgins, heartless repudiations of childless women, and forced marriages between adolescent girls and 50-year-old men. One might be tempted to question the author/narrator's purpose in recounting these "horror stories" in a publication that is obviously destined for Western audiences. I do not suggest that Djura herself has not suffered at the hands of her family and society. She is no doubt, as her autobiography reveals, a woman who has had to persevere and display more courage and determination than many women will ever need to in order to achieve their goals.

My concern in reading her narrative is that as both a popular entertainer and now an author, Djura has come to occupy a position as a kind of spokesperson for North African women in France. Yet what can her account contribute to a spirit of reconciliation and tolerance between the ideals of French society and the images associated with north African cultures? The only positive portrayal of North African culture in her account involves Kabyle music and oral poetry. It is clear that it is to France and to the benefits of having grown up and been educated in France that Djura attributes her survival, her personal liberation, and her success. This work then, can be read as a hymn to the integration and assimilation of north African women into French society. *Le Voile du silence* places itself squarely into the double-bind paradigm of "tradition" versus "modernity." Abdelkrim-Chikh's (1991) study of exogamous marriage among North African women in France has identified the same dilemma as a common concern among many second-generation Maghrebian women. All too often *integration* means "wearing the same uniform as everyone else" (p. 244). The idea of modernity blended with tradition, rather than modernity in place of tradition surfaces with difficulty in such a climate.

What this means for north African women in France is that they fight a daily battle to prove that it is not "France" that has "liberated" them, but rather the women themselves who have struggled within their own culture as well as within French society to impose themselves as subjects acting of their own free will. One of Abdelkrim-Chikh's (1991) consultants summed up this problem when she related that French society is eager to take the credit for a personal liberation that was the individual women's own doing:

> At the start of your rebellion, you are angry and you cry out and they (the sociologists and journalists), they are more than happy to latch onto the negative and they don't need to know any more than that, since we are the ones telling them everything they want to hear; they are happy and they don't listen beyond that, they just want to hear that our parents are backward SOBs and they don't even check to see if it's true. (p. 245)

Here I briefly contrast Nedjma Plantade's *L'Honneur et l'amertume* with Djura's *Le Voile du silence*. Plantade's transcribed oral autobiography of Louisa Azzizen closely follows the model that Lazreg (1988) has suggested is particularly valuable in understanding Algerian women's reality. It is a narrative that attempts to go beyond the common paradigm of accounts of Arab women's victimization at the hands of their menfolk and their society. *L'Honneur et l'amertume* presents what Lazreg would term the "lived reality. . . . The Algerian woman as a subject in her own right" (p. 94). Plantade (1993), an anthropologist by training, informed the reader in her preface that her objective in transcribing Louisa Azzizen's oral life history is to provide second- or third-generation Franco-Algerians with a portrait of a woman whose voice and whose story history might otherwise have forgotten. She stated that in Azzizen:

> young French people who are themselves a product of Algerian immigration, in a legitimate search for their past, may discover or rediscover the image of their mother or grandmother—silent wives of worn out husbands who have never disturbed France—but who might have given birth to a sometimes noisy generation. (p. 13)

Her intended audience then, is not a Western reader avid for a description of women's oppression. Louisa Azzizen's story is meant to further the cause of tolerance and understanding between first-generation north African immigrants and their offspring. The fact that French readers may also gain invaluable insight into understanding the "lived reality" of an illiterate Kabyle-Algerian woman is a welcome bonus.

Azzizen's story begins in a mountain village of Kabylia. Her descriptions of the first several decades of her life portray many pleasurable episodes: holidays, childhood games, and family gatherings. Her life changed after marriage to a boy from a large farming family. Louisa Azzizen's life is then a tale of hardship: poverty, hard work, and the inevitable difficulties of dealing with her in-laws. Plantade (1993) arranged the oral interview into an account that explains potentially unfamiliar cultural practices in footnotes. Her transcription of Louisa Azzizen's narrative demonstrates a clear concern for the cultural and socioreligious context of her consultant's story. In 1960, Azzizen's husband took her and their first four children to France. The remaining sections of her narrative detail the difficulties she experienced as a new immigrant in Paris, uncertain how to negotiate the obstacles she confronted in this new life in France. These new challenges included desperate living conditions, the children's schooling, medical exams including childbirth in an unaccustomed physical position, and visits from a French social worker.

Her new life in France pleased her, despite the uncertainties. Azzizen's narrative ends on a tone of hope for the future of her children in France. She and her husband tried their best to understand the new ideas brought home by the children—especially their daughters' demands to remain in school and train for careers outside the home. In her oral account, Louisa Azzizen emphasized that what upset her most was what she perceived to be a common French attitude that Algerian immigrants are somehow "ungrateful" for the life and the advantages they discovered in France. She concluded the account of her life with the observation that Algerian immigrants of her generation, women and men alike, have only scratched the surface of understanding France and its civilization; their generation has been sacrificed, ignored in their exile both by Algeria and France. She observed:

> In reality, France, this nation that Algerians continue to dream about, is only good for those who know it well, those who can come here and be like a fish in water. But for the poor folk like us, France will always be inaccessible. Only our children, and that's for the best, will maybe be able to live full lives here, those who have grown up here, who have been caught up in material things, education, comfort, and above all, liberty, this strange idea that for many years seemed so shocking to me and yet today I have somehow managed to accept without even knowing how. . . . (p. 265)

The future for north African women immigrants and their daughters in France will ultimately result from individual personal choices and much intercultural negotiation. All of us, Western readers as well as Maghrebian women in France themselves, could benefit by moving beyond reduction of the cultural "Other" to an essentializing difference, even if such reactions result from well-intentioned concern for women's rights and living conditions. There is no monolithic reality for Maghrebian women either in France or in North Africa. Each woman "speaks for" herself and seeks solutions to the many issues confronting her; although these choices might provide a model for others, ultimately, every woman's "coming to the word," to paraphrase Hélène Cixous (1977), is her own right and responsibility. For those with no access to *la parole*, the temptation to "speak for others" should be avoided. I see Nedjma Plantade's example of "facilitating" a woman's (Louisa Azzizen's) access to the written word as ultimately resulting in more useful outcomes than Djura's work. It is Djura's stated desire to raise the "veil of silence" for other north African women I find problematic. I honor her choice to tell of her own story, but my conviction that each individual's voice speaks for itself leads me to resist its generalization to become the voice of others. We benefit from hearing voices of both Djura and Louisa Azzizen, yet we need to keep in mind for whom, and to whom they speak.

REFERENCES

Abdelkrim-Chikh, R. (1991). Les Femmes exogames: Entre la loi de dieu et les droits de l'homme [Exogamous women: Between God's law and human rights]. In B. Etienne (Ed.), *L'Islam en France* [Islam in France] (pp. 235-254). Paris: Editions du CNRS.

Begag, A., & Chaouite, A. (1990). *Ecarts d'identité* [Identity gaps]. Paris: Seuil.

Bernard, P. (1993). *L'immigration* [Immigration]. Paris: Editions Le Monde.

Cixous, H. (1977). La venue à l'écriture. In H. Cixous, M. Gagnon, & A. Leclerc (Eds.), *La venue à l'écriture* (pp. 9-62). Paris: Union Générale d'Editions.

Djura. (1990). *Le Voile du silence* [The veil of silence]. Paris: Michel Lafon.

Etienne, B. (1991). *L'Islam en France* [Islam in France]. Paris: Ed. du CNRS.

Lazreg, M. (1988). Feminism and difference: The perils of writing as a woman on women in Algeria. *Feminist Studies, 14*(1), 81-107.

Mermet, G. (1992). *Francoscopie 1993*. Paris: Larousse.

Mohanty, C. T. (1991). Under western eyes: Feminist scholarship and colonial discourses. In C. T. Mohanty, A. Russo, & L. Torres (Eds.), *Third world women and the politics of feminism* (pp. 51-80). Bloomington: University of Indiana Press.

Naïr, S. (1992). *Le Regard des vainqueurs: Les enjeux Français de l'immigration* [The gaze of the conquerors: French immigration dilemmas]. Paris: Bernard Grasset.

Plantade, N. (1993). *L'Honneur et l'amertume: Le destin ordinaire d'une femme Kabyle* [Honor and bitterness: The normal fate of a Kabyle woman]. Paris: Balland.

Spivak, G. (1980). Poststructuralism, marginality, postcoloniality, and value. In P. Collier & H. Geyer-Ryan (Eds.), *Literary theory today* (pp. 219-244). Ithaca, NY: Cornell University Press.

Spivak, G. (1988). Can the subaltern speak? In C. Nelson & L. Grossberg (Eds.), *Marxism and the interpretation of culture* (pp. 271-313). Chicago: University of Chicago Press.

13

HOMELESS WOMEN'S INNER VOICES: FRIENDS OR FOES?

DOMINIQUE M. GENDRIN

We are [. . . .] not involved in the study of social communication and
social justice; we haven't even put our toe in the shallow end of this
very large pool. This is clearly a shame, for I believe that we have much
to say that could be helpful to [the poor, the homeless, the aged, the
abused]. Social justice is most certainly a communication issue, for it is
constituted in the pattern of interaction in which social actors in a
system engage. (Frey, 1994, p. 8)

One of the fastest growing segments of the homeless population has
been families (i.e., women with children and couples with children;
Waxman & Reyes, 1987). Often referred to as the *new homeless*, this
particular group is at risk of homelessness because of a change in
circumstances, such as unemployment, spousal abuse, and/or eviction.
However, little research has focused primarily or exclusively on
homeless women (Hagen, 1990). Furthermore, no studies have been
conducted thus far on the intrapersonal communication dimension of
homelessness (Gendrin, 1993a, 1993b).

This chapter focuses on the inner voices of homeless women as mental representations of their homeless social experiences. Inner voices take the form of internal dialogues, a thought process associated with the internal transformation of communication systems among social groups marginal to mainstream society (Edwards, Honeycutt, & Zagacki, 1988; Gendrin, 1993a). Internal dialogues take place with significant others about current relational issues. They represent one cognitive activity by which women and men process social experience. Not only do internal dialogues promote social and psychological well-being, they also contribute to women's and men's social competence (Honeycutt, 1989, 1992). Yet, when women and men experience loneliness, they report less internal communication activity, imagine themselves in conversations that are different from actual ones, and dialogue internally with fewer relational partners.

Although internal dialogues guide how women and men think about relationships, as well as how they perceive, evaluate, recall, and edit ongoing interactions with others (Honeycutt, 1993), how this mental activity is affected when women and men experience homelessness is not known. Homelessness, a unique social experience associated with a lack of social support, can generate a sense of hopelessness and helplessness. Considering that social isolation impacts social and psychological well-being, learning the impact of homelessness on homeless women's ability to process social experience is important. Hence, the purpose of this chapter is twofold: First, it presents the results of a study examining the features of homeless women's internal dialogues in relation to their social experience, and second, it listens to some of the homeless women's "inner voices" in the form of actual lines of dialogues they imagine having with the people in their lives.

HOMELESS WOMEN

Few studies have focused on the unique characteristics and needs of women experiencing homelessness. Studies of homelessness among families have revealed some important factors associated with homelessness among women. Structural factors, such as poor economic conditions and lack of low-income housing (Elliott & Krivo, 1991; McChesney, 1990, 1993), as well as individual factors, such as mental illness or alcohol or drug abuse (see Fischer & Breakey, 1991; Goodman, Saxe, & Harvey, 1991) have put women at risk of becoming homeless. Women at risk of being homeless are most often mothers, are under the age of 35, are members of a minority group, have often not completed high school, and have usually experienced more than one episode of homelessness (Milburn & Booth, 1990).

The characteristics of homelessness also reveal several gender differences (Hagen, 1990). Homeless women are somewhat more likely than homeless men to be mentally ill, but they are less likely than homeless men to experience difficulties with alcohol and drug abuse. In a critical review of the research on homeless families since 1980, McChesney (1993) summarized the risk factors of homelessness as: the shortage of affordable housing, single-mother families, minority families, young maternal age, substance abuse, domestic violence, pregnancy, and the size and proximity of a support network of family members and friends.

Disaffiliation from family, friends, and social roles is an important characteristic of homeless women. However, for women with children, disaffiliation may be experienced somewhat differently. According to Crystal (1984), homeless women maintain some kind of parental relationship regardless of whether they have their children with them. Additionally, many women report having close personal relationships (Hagen & Ivanoff, 1988). The more recent literature on the subject argues that a failure in the support systems of women already at risk is an important cause for homelessness (Grisby, Baumann, Gregorich, & Roberts-Gray, 1990). Concurrently, friends and relatives may serve as safety nets in preventing homelessness (Milburn & D'Ercole, 1991a).

HOMELESS WOMEN'S INNER VOICES

The study of homeless women's inner voices is based on the notion that individuals experience some internal disequilibrium when they feel out of place within the larger social environment (Gendrin, 1993a). Homeless women experience a breakdown of their meaning systems because they have lost most, if not all, modes of social identification. Not only are they without a home, but they have also lost their sense of self as workers, friends, caregivers, and family members (Goodman et al., 1991). With the loss of one's place in society comes the disintegration of relational expectancies, communication rules, and behaviors associated with being a functional member of society.

What homeless women do, think, and feel cannot be explained without understanding the way they construct reality in their minds. Because social isolation is both a cause and consequence of homelessness, it is important to examine the impact of social isolation on relational thought processes and more specifically, the type of disruption it creates about knowledge structures regarding homeless women's relationships. Understanding the nature of homeless women's internal dialogues offers insight into the way they process their experience and into the impact their new social experience has on their mental health (Edwards et al., 1988).

Research on the social support available to homeless women points to various interaction partners, such as their own children, other homeless shelter residents, friends, and relatives who are living in distant communities. According to Honeycutt (1993), long distance relationships can also be maintained through internal dialogues with the absent partner. Knowing the relational partners with whom the homeless women imagine themselves conversing will help determine the extent to which they review current relational experiences as well as relive past relationships. Honeycutt (1989) suggested that internal dialogues help women sort out their expectations and interpretations of past events and encounters as well as future ones. For homeless women, this mental activity could compensate for the lack of a sufficient support system of friends and relatives.

Another feature of internal dialogues involves topics of conversations that reflect current, as well as past, life issues. Yet it is not known about what homeless women imagine conversing. It is reasonable to assume that they might review in their minds relationships that have turned sour, due to family violence, eviction by landlords, spousal abuse, or divorce. They may converse mentally about their predicament, such as a lack of money, interpersonal conflict, loss of housing. Identifying the topical nature of homeless women's internal dialogues would clarify the extent to which internal dialogues promote a tenuous sense of well-being or influence homeless women in mulling about hard times.

HOMELESS WOMEN AND SOCIAL ISOLATION

Researchers argue that women and men are psychologically and physically healthy to the extent that their means of communication enable them to function effectively in their surroundings (Kim, 1988; Ruesch, 1951/1968). Homeless women often see their network of friends and relatives disappear and their opportunities for interaction as full members of the larger community diminish dramatically. When they lack a support system, homeless women experience great mental and physical handicaps (see, e.g., Cohen & Wills, 1985).

Loneliness has been associated with low-income groups, the psychiatrically impaired, and highly stressed populations (see Rook, 1988, for a review of the research on loneliness among various groups). Although loneliness can be considered a dispositional characteristic for some women (see Shaver, Furnam, & Buhrmester, 1985), the use of loneliness as a measure of social isolation in this study is based on the notion that it is enhanced by structural and environmental factors (see Peplau & Perlman, 1982), such as those associated with homelessness. When reviewing the research on social isolation among homeless women, Crystal (1984) reported that women with children residing in shelters experience a different type of disaffiliation from other homeless women because they maintain some type of parental relationship with their children, maintaining in the process the vital link between family members.

Loneliness is of theoretical importance in the present study because empirical evidence shows its negative impact on women's ability to activate an appropriate relational script for actual encounters. In a review of the research on social relationships and loneliness, Berg and Piner (1989) concluded that the means to ward off loneliness and be psychologically healthy is to be able to maintain a satisfying network of friends or relatives. Yet, it is not known whether homeless women experience satisfying relationships nor the extent to which these relationships ward off a sense of loneliness.

METHODOLOGY

This study selected the marginal housing definition of homelessness for two reasons: First, it refers to persons in transitional shelters who are, overwhelmingly, women; and second, such women are least likely to report recent alcohol and both lifetime and recent illicit drug use (see Johnson, Mitra, Newman, & Horm, 1993, for a review of the various definitions of homelessness). These two criteria for sampling selection made it easier to focus on a subgroup of homeless women with no history of alcohol or drug use, a factor that could have influenced the validity of the findings.

Over a period of 1 year, 75 residents of a women's shelter located in a medium size community in the south participated in the study. The shelter was in an apartment complex and only accepted women residents with young children. To stay at the shelter, one could not have a recent history of alcohol and/or drug use. The majority of the women were single, the others were either divorced, separated, or widowed. They had between one and two children, had been homeless between 1 month and 8 years, and their educational levels varied between sixth grade and 2 years of college. Although a convenience sample, the group of homeless women who served as subjects for the study was representative of the population of homeless women in the area (see Curol & Foster, 1993).[1]

The questionnaire included four standardized instruments: the Relationship Satisfaction Survey, the Survey of Internal dialogues, the UCLA Loneliness Scale, and the Measurement of Life Satisfaction. The format, wording, and length of the questions asked raised some methodological problems that were addressed in the following way. Because of concern that the format, length, and wording of the questionnaire might discourage the respondents, the questionnaire was orally administered. Doing so also helped establish a personal rapport with the respondents.[2] The interviewer was trained to provide consistent answers if points of clarification were needed. Wording of the Survey of Internal Conversations instrument was modified after testing it on a small sample of homeless women. Specifically, the expression "imagined conversations" used in the original survey produced a negative, emotional reaction by respondents, such as: "Oh, I don't imagine things!" Therefore, the expression "imagined conversations" was replaced with "internal conversations."

Survey of Internal Conversations. The survey used included 39 close-ended statements evaluated on a 7-point scale. Honeycutt and his colleagues (1990) identified eight imagined conversation characteristics. The characteristics were as follows: activity ("I often have internal conversations"), pleasantness ("My internal conversations are pleasant/unpleasant"), discrepancy ("My internal conversations are dissimilar to actual conversations"), self-dominance ("I speak more than my partner(s) in my internal conversations"), proactivity ("My internal conversations precede actual encounters"), retroactivity ("My internal conversations follow actual conversations"), specificity ("My internal conversations are very specific"). Two open-ended questions asked respondents to list some of the topics they recently discussed in their internal dialogues, and the relational partners with whom they had the most internal conversations. Respondents could also report actual lines of conversations they recently imagined having with their partners.[3]

---

[1]The subjects ranged between ages 18 and 53 (M = 34); they had between one and two children (M = 1.21); they had been homeless between 1 month and 8 years (M = 21.24 months); and had an educational level that varied between Grade 6 and 2 years of college.

[2]The author would like to thank Catherine Bonds for conducting the interviews. Catherine is an undergraduate student in communication studies at McNeese State University in Lake Charles, Louisianna.

[3]The reliability estimates for the eight dimensions were as follows: activity (Cronbach α = .69); pleasantness (Cronbach α = .69); variety (Cronbach α = .57);

Measure of Life Satisfaction. This survey (Neugarten, Havighurst, & Tobin, 1961) included two parts. Index A included 20 statements concerning life in general. Respondents either "agreed," "disagreed" or "did not know." Some of the items were "This is the dreariest time of my life," " I expect some interesting and pleasant things to happen to me in the future," "I would not change my past even if I could." Six open-ended questions made up Index B . The questions addressed specific issues, such as the future, the most important thing in life right now, loneliness, and a satisfying way of life.[4]

Although the survey was derived from a measure of life satisfaction for the elderly, the questions about various life changes were general enough that they were applicable to different social groups. Furthermore, none of the items asked explicitly about the respondents' moods or psychological health, but the items that asked about the most important thing in life right now, loneliness, and a satisfying way of life, were thought to reflect a general perception about life stressors.

UCLA Loneliness Scale. The revised UCLA Loneliness Scale served as a measure of social isolation (Russell, Peplau, & Cutrona, 1980). The scale includes 20 items using a 4-point scale (1 = never; 2 = rarely; 3 = sometimes; 4 = often).[5] The items measured satisfaction and dissatisfaction with social relationships. For example, " I lack companionship," "I am no longer close to anyone," and "l am unhappy being so withdrawn."

Relationship Satisfaction Survey. The Relationship Satisfaction Survey (Hendrick, 1981) first asked about the person(s) to whom the respondent talked to the most. The next six questions were closed-end questions on a 5-point scale, asking about the respondent's level of

---

discrepancy (Cronbach α = .78); self-dominance (Cronbach α = .80); proactivity (Cronbach α = .80); retroactivity (Cronbach α = .77); specificity (Cronbach α = .51). Honeycutt and his colleagues reported higher reliability estimates for the eight dimensions of internal dialogues: activity (Cronbach α = .84); pleasantness (Cronbach α = .84); discrepancy (Cronbach α = .86); self-dominance (Cronbach α = .77); proactivity (Cronbach α = .80); retroactivity (Cronbach α = .73); specificity (Cronbach α = .77) (Honeycutt et al., 1989-1990; Zagacki et al., 1992).

[4]The combined correlation coefficient score for both indexes was .73 (N = 91) Neugarten, Havighurst, & Tobin, 1961; Index A (Cronbach α = .75); Index B (Cronbach α = .67).

[5]The combined correlation coefficient score for the two indexes was .86 (p < .000). The internal consistency of the revised scale was .94 (Russell, Peplau, & Cutrona, 1980).

satisfaction with various characteristics of their relationships. For example, "In general, how satisfied are you with these relationships?" and "How satisfied are you with how your relationships compare with other women's relationships?"[6]

RESULTS

The relational partners and topics of conversation homeless women reported in their internal dialogues were categorized using inductive analysis. One undergraduate student assisted the experimenter in developing the categories and two other undergraduate coders coded the data.[7]

Relational Partners. The categories were derived in part from the category systems developed by Edwards et al. (1988) and Honeycutt (1989). Relational partners were coded into seven categories: roommates, family members, spiritual leaders, women in authority, friends, romantic partners, and others. Homeless women imagined themselves conversing with partners in each category.[8]

Topics Imagined. Topics of conversations imagined by homeless women were coded into 13 categories: health matters, general life issues, religion, interpersonal conflict, money, past events, relationships, feelings, work, sex, future goals, education, and abuse. The topics included:

1. Relationships (e.g., family, friends, ex-husband).
2. Money.
3. Work.
4. Future goals (e.g., moving on, getting a house, getting married, getting help, getting the children again).
5. General life issues (e.g., quality of life, discrimination, raising children, being homeless).

---

[6]The Hendrick's (1981) Relationship Assessment Scale from which the Relationship Satisfaction Scale is derived showed a Cronbach's α of .71.

[7]Intercoder level of agreement for imagined interaction topics was .94, and for imagined interaction partners, the level of agreement was .91 (Holsti, 1968).

[8]The imagined relational partners with whom homeless women imagined themselves conversing were family members (34.5%), romantic partners (21.5%), friends (16.8%), spiritual leaders (10%; e.g. pastor of the shelter, God), roommates (6.5%), women in authority (2.8%; e.g., employers, landlords).

6. Religion (God, church).
7. Abuse (e.g., child abuse and alcohol and drug abuse).
8. Interpersonal conflict (e.g., marriage problems, disagreement with other shelter residents).
9. Feelings (e.g., jealousy, fear, resentment).
10. Past events (e.g., growing up, home/life the way it used to be).
11. Miscellaneous.
12. Health issues (e.g., getting sick; finding a nurse for a sick child).
13. Education.
14. Sex.[9]

In order to put homeless women's imagined conversational partners and topics into perspective, the homeless women in this study were asked to write actual lines of dialogues reflecting their most recent internal conversations.

Internal Conversations. Of the 75 homeless women, 35 gave scripts of their internal dialogues. To understand their concerns it is useful to see the exact words.

Many of these dialogues focus on relationships with ex-husbands, fiances, boyfriends, fathers of the children who were "absent" because the shelter only accepted women and children, or who left when the family became homeless. The extent to which the conversations feature these men reflects how important such relationships (and the often resulting conflicts) are to these women. The following conversation about such a man is typical.

—Larry is not for real/. He tells you one thing. You deserve better. . . . Think of your kids.
—I like Larry.
—I know.

---

[9]Imagined interaction topics included: relationships (23.5%; e.g., family, friends, ex-husband), money (12.5%), work (10%), future goals (10%; e.g., moving on, getting a house, getting married, getting help, getting the children again), general life issues (7%; e.g., quality of life, discrimination, raising children, being homeless), religion (7%; God, church), abuse (5.7%; e.g., child abuse and alcohol and drug abuse), interpersonal conflict (5%; e.g., marriage problems, disagreement with other shelter residents), feelings (4.7%; e.g., jealousy, fear, resentment), past events (3.8%; e.g., growing up, home/life the way it used to be), miscellaneous (3%), health issues (2%; e.g., getting sick; finding a nurse for my little girl), education (2%), and sex (2%).

Others of the imagined conversations reflected the abusive nature of the relationships between some homeless women and their male partners:

—*Either be a father or a payment!*
—*Go to hell! I won't do either*

—*I hate you!*
—*I'd rather see you dead than free from me!*

Many of the internal conversations were with the absent male partner. The following dialogue between a homeless woman and her absent male partner focused on the absence of the father from the children's lives and the reasons she imagines him giving.

—*You think I'm not a good mother. I'm the one here [at the shelter].*
—*You know how it is. How hard it is for a black man.*

Other conversations point out the importance of parenting to the homeless women.

—*Yes, I do [think my kids are important]. They go before my husband.*
—*You care more about the kids than me.*

Many of the dialogues reflect the women's desire to maintain the relationship with the absent man, as in the following conversation with a roommate about the homeless woman's ex-husband and how she might get him back.

—*Why did he leave me?*
—*I don't know.*
—*I need a job and a better place to live and he might come back.*
—*Maybe.*
—*I wish he would come back.*

Another woman expresses a similar point, this one with less focus on her own causal role.

—*Why hasn't he called, or written me, or anything. He won't accept my call.*
—*Don't want to be bothered.*
—*He felt guilty because he walked out on them [the children].*

Some of the internal conversations reflect the women's less positive feelings about men, as this one with a roommate.

—*They want you to go out and drink with them, but don't get drunk. . . . If you get drunk, then, you can't take care of them.*
—*But drunk enough to have sex.*

Another such exchange imagines talking to the drinking man himself.

—*You been drinking*
—*but I thought you were pregnant*
—*I'm not sure if I am or not. But even if I am, what does it matter to you!*
—*Well, if it's mine. The way you are acting, you don't really care.*

Other internal dialogues focus on alcohol addiction and recovery. In the first exchange, a homeless woman reports her ideas of an intervention in another homeless woman's problem.

—*I don't know. My friend wants to recover and she has an addiction.*
—*She needs bible scriptures read to her from the bible and watch biblical tapes. Get a hypnotist before to get her to forget her past and get on with the future.*

The dialogues often suggest hope of getting out of homelessness. One woman engaged such a conversation with God; the other talked with a roommate.

—*God, please protect my children*
—*Have no fear.*

—*I went job hunting today.*
—*Any luck?*
—*I turned in a couple of applications.*
—*Maybe they'll pan out.*

Sometimes the focus was on other concerns. The following imagined conversation with the pastor of the shelter about a woman's concern that she might have been seen by someone from her hometown was one such case.

—*I had known the girl. She might let someone know I was here.*
—*I should talk to her and tell her the situation.*

Even in these concerns, however, relationships often figured prominently. The following dialogue with a roommate illustrates:

—You should not blame yourself for your mom being in a nursing home.
—I should have brought her a home. She would never have done this to me.

Memories of the past were also among the topics of the women's internal dialogues, although these, too, often involved relationships.

—I wished I had land to plant my own garden.
—That would be nice. I am too old for this now

—Well, Sis, I wished you had not left Maine.
—It is so hot and humid here.
—It is sad not to see each other much now.

—Mom, I really miss my childhood.
—I understand, but you can't go back to that
—But I want to . . .

Homeless women's inner voices reflect longing for a happier past or a better future, talk of the pain of broken relationships, addiction, and abuse. Some voices come from the past and some from the present. They link homeless women to a life of continuity and change. But consistently, the internal dialogues show the maintenance function they perform for relationships and, perhaps as a result, general life satisfaction. Although the relationship was a weak one, homeless women's level of satisfaction with their current relationships was positively related to an overall measure of life satisfaction.[10] A lack of specificity in homeless women's internal dialogues was the only evidence of the impact of loneliness in their lives.[11]

---

[10]The relation between homeless women's life satisfaction, relationship satisfaction, and loneliness was measured using Pearson correlations. Both Life Satisfaction indexes correlated significantly with relationship satisfaction (Index A: $r = .32$; Index B: $r = .25$). The Relationship Satisfaction Scale scores were correlated with scores on the UCLA Loneliness Scale using two-tailed levels of significance. There may be a weak negative relation between relationship satisfaction and loneliness; however, the correlation did not achieve statistical significance ($r = -.20$, $p = .078$). The correlation between loneliness and the first Life Satisfaction index did not show a significant correlation (Index A: $r = -.18$). There was a significant negative relationship between loneliness and the second Life Satisfaction Index (Index B: $r = -.27$).

[11]The third research question examined the relation between homeless women's loneliness and their imagined interaction characteristics. Pearson correlations revealed a negative relation between loneliness and specificity ($r = -.30$). The relations between loneliness and other internal dialogue characteristics were not significant.

DISCUSSION

This study provided some useful information about the intrapersonal communication dimension of transitional homelessness among women. First, an examination of internal dialogue partners and topics of conversation revealed the importance of relationships in the lives and minds of homeless women. More than half of the imagined interactional partners were family members, romantic partners or friends. Relationships also dominated the topics of conversations imagined by homeless women. This feature of homeless women's internal conversations supports the relational maintenance function of internal dialogues. For homeless women, imagining themselves in conversations with close ones enables them to maintain a sense of social connectedness that may help compensate for actual encounters. Thinking and talking internally about relationships allows homeless women to review or rewrite scripts for past and future conversations. This mental activity serves to make sense of their social experiences.

In examining the other topics discussed in homeless women's internal dialogues, results revealed internal conversations about money, work, and future goals, such as getting a house of their own, moving on, getting a job. This other feature of homeless women's internal dialogues illustrates the function internal dialogues perform in constructing one's social reality (Honeycutt, 1989). Homeless women's inner voices were the means to envision the kind of life they will have when they are able to leave the shelter and be economically and socially self-sufficient. Thus, these inner voices function to assist in the homeless women's construction of social reality.

It is interesting to note that the homeless women in this study did not report a strong sense of social isolation. Studies on homelessness consistently identify social isolation and a lack of social support as both a cause and consequence of homelessness. Yet the study reported a positive relation between life satisfaction and relationship satisfaction. The only impact of homeless women's feeling of loneliness was their limited ability to recall specific lines of dialogues. Despite their restricted social life, homeless women were able to derive satisfaction in their ongoing relationships and, consequently, did not experience the loneliness associated with losing relational partners. Additionally, it is reasonable to assume that women with whom they are in contact, such as other homeless women, shelter pastors, and female relatives and friends, provide them with necessary emotional support. Furthermore, most of the homeless women participating in this study had children with them. Because they are able to maintain a parental role, homeless mothers experience less estrangement than their childless counterparts, and may be compelled to maintain a sense of normalcy in their relationships for the sake of the children. Finally, the shelter was located in an apartment complex, which may have promoted a sense of leading a fairly normal life despite the overwhelming magnitude of the problems they have to face.

Homeless women's level of loneliness had little impact on their thought processes about relationships. The only discrepancy in their internal dialogues, in comparison to other populations, was that they showed little specificity. Research has shown that when internal dialogues are negatively related to loneliness, women experience low mental health (Edwards et al., 1988; Honeycutt, Edwards, & Zagacki, 1989-1990). This study indicates, on the other hand, that homeless women's inner voices contribute to their mental health. These results confirm the findings that homeless mothers residing in shelters report an overall good psychosocial well-being (Dail, 1990). Although greater loneliness would lead to the disruption of homeless women's internal communication systems, transitional homelessness may only set women on the outer boundaries of their social worlds, never quite outcasts, although removed enough from mainstream society to be at risk of becoming total strangers.

This study suggests some ideas for both further research and for practice. We need to gather data examining the relation between the functions of internal dialogues and homeless women's psychological well-being. In particular, we need to learn how internal dialogues function to relieve tension and negative feelings, generate greater self-understanding, and help sort out one's inner thoughts. That homelessness is a critical experience in one's life that would trigger greater mental activity in comparison to women who enjoy the safety and security of a home and a job is a reasonable hypothesis. If so, homeless women's internal dialogue functions may differ qualitatively and quantitatively from those of nonhomeless women. Another step to take in understanding the disruption homelessness creates in women's lives would be to examine the characteristics and functions of internal dialogues in relation to impact on homeless women's communication competence. Honeycutt et al. (1992) reported a significant relation between the rehearsal, planning, and review functions of internal dialogues and communication competence. Also worth examining would be gender differences in homelessness. Loneliness research suggests that women and men experience homelessness differently (Berg & Piner, 1989). Loneliness among homeless men is defined in terms of social isolation, whereas homeless women experience emotional isolation. It might be possible to argue that loneliness could have a differing impact on homeless women's and men's imagined interaction characteristics and functions, creating in the process varying disruption in their internal communication systems.

Finally, this study has demonstrated at least one important idea for application in working with homeless women. It has provided some evidence illustrating the supportive function of homeless women's inner voices as the women transit through a shelter system. In this regard, the mental activity of internal dialogue has been helpful in sustaining a sense of psychological and social well-being for homeless women. Persons working in social service roles with homeless women in settings such as the one described here should promote opportunities for internal conversations. By so doing they would take one small step in avoiding the desperation and learned helplessness that sometimes come with homelessness.

REFERENCES

Berg, J. H., & Piner, K. E. (1989). Social relationships and the lack of social relationships. In S. Duck with R. Cohen Silver (Ed.), *Personal relationships and social support* (pp. 140-158). Newbury Park, CA: Sage.

Cohen, S., & Wills, T. A. (1985). Stress, social support, and the buffering hypothesis. *Psychological Bulletin, 98*, 310-357.

Crystal, S. (1984). Homeless men and homeless women: The gender gap. *Urban and Social Change Review, 17*, 2-6.

Curol, H., & Foster, D. (1993, March). *Local research: Its value and validity in studying homelessness among women.* Paper presented at the 1994 South Central Women's Studies Association Conference, New Orleans, LA.

Dail, P. W. (1990). The psychosocial context of homeless mothers with young children: Program and policy implications. *Child Welfare League of America, 54*, 291-308.

Edwards, R., Honeycutt, J. M., & Zagacki, K. S. (1988). Imagined interaction as an element of social cognition. *Western Journal of Speech Communication, 52*, 23-45.

Elliott, M., & Krivo, L. J. (1991). Structural determinants of homelessness in the United States. *Social Problems, 38*, 113-131.

Fischer, P. J., & Breakey, W. R. (1991). The epidemiology of alcohol, drug, and mental disorders among homeless persons. *American Psychologist, 46*, 1115-1128.

Frey, L. (1994, August). *Communication and social justice: The search for the Holy Grail or looking for justice in all the wrong places.* Keynote address presented at the Institute for Faculty Development: Theory and Research, Holland, MI.

Gendrin, D. (1993a, November). *Homelessness: A communication perspective*. Paper presented at the annual Speech Communication Association Convention, Miami, FL.

Gendrin, D. (1993b, November). *Internal dialogues among homeless people: Friends or foes?* Paper presented at the annual Speech Communication Association Convention, Miami, FL.

Goodman, L., Saxe, L., & Harvey, M. (1991). Homelessness as psychological trauma: Broadening perspectives. *American Psychologist, 46*, 1219-1225.

Grisby, C., Baumann, D., Gregorich, S.E., & Roberts-Gray, C. (1990). Disaffiliation to entrenchment: A model for understanding homelessness. *Journal of Social Issues, 46*, 141-156.

Hagen, J. L. (1990). Designing services for homeless women. *Journal of Health and Social Policy, 1*, 1-15.

Hagen, J. L., & Ivanoff, A. M. (1988). Homeless women: A high risk population. *Affilia, 3*(1), 19-33.

Hendrick, S. S. (1981). Self-disclosure and marital satisfaction. *Journal of Personality and Social Psychology, 40*, 1150-1159.

Holsti, O. R. (1969). *Content analysis for the social sciences and humanitites*. Reading, MA: Addison-Wesley.

Honeycutt, J. M. (1989). A functional analysis of imagined interaction activity in everyday life. In J. E. Shorr, P. Robin, J. A. Connella, & M. Wolpin (Eds.), *Imagery: Current perspectives* (pp. 13-26). New York: Plenum Press.

Honeycutt, J. M. (1993). Memory structures for the rise and fall of personal relationships. In S. Duck (Ed.), *Individuals in relationships: Women in relationships* (pp. 60-86). Newbury Park, CA: Sage.

Honeycutt, J. M., Edwards, R., & Zagacki, K. S. (1989-1990). Using imagined interaction features to predict measures of self-awareness: Loneliness, locus of control, self-dominance, and emotional intensity. *Imagination, Cognition and Personality, 9*, 17-31.

Honeycutt, J. M., Zagacki, K. S., & Edwards, R. (1990). Imagined interaction and interpersonal communication. *Communication Reports, 3*, 1-8

Honeycutt, J. M., Zagacki, K. S., & Edwards, R. (1992). Imagined interaction, conversational sensitivity and communication competence. *Imagination, Cognition and Personality, 12*, 139-157.

Johnson, T. P., Mitra, A., Newman, R., & Horm, J. (1993). Problems of definition in sampling special populations: The case of homeless persons. *Evaluation Practice, 14*, 119-126.

Kim, Y. Y. (1988). *Communication and cross-cultural adaptation: An integrative theory*. Clevedon: Multilingual Matters LTD.

McChesney, K. Y. (1990). Family homelessness: A systemic problem. *Journal of Social Issues, 46,* 191-205.

McChesney, K. Y. (1993). Homeless families since 1980: Implications for education. *Education and Urban Society, 25,* 361-380.

Milburn, N., & Booth, J. (1990). Sociodemographic, homeless state and mental health characteristics of women in shelters: Preliminary findings. *Urban Research Review, 12*(2), 104.

Milburn, N., & D'Ercole, A. (1991a). Homeless women: Moving toward a comprehensive model. *American Psychologist, 46,* 1161-1169.

Milburn, N., & D'Ercole, A. (1991b). Homeless women, children, and families. *American Psychologist, 46,* 1159-1160.

Neugarten, B. L., Havighurst, R. J., & Tobin, S. E. (1961). The measurement of life satisfaction. *Journal of Gerontology, 16,* 134-143.

Peplau, L. A., & Perlman, D. (Eds.). (1982). *Loneliness: A sourcebook of current theory, research and therapy.* New York: Wiley-Interscience.

Rook, K. S. (1988). Toward a more differentiated view of loneliness. In S. W. Duck (Ed.), *Handbook of personal relationships* (pp. 571-589). London: John Wiley.

Ruesch, J. (1968). Communication and human relations: An interdisciplinary approach. In J. Ruesch & G. Bateson (Eds.), *Communication: The social matrix of psychiatry* (pp. 21-49). New York: Norton. (Original work published 1951)

Russell, D., Peplau, L. A., & Cutrona, C. E. (1980). The revised UCLA loneliness scale: Concurrent and discriminant validity evidence. *Journal of Personality and Social Psychology, 39,* 472-480.

Shaver, P., Furnam, W., & Buhrmester, D. (1985). Aspects of a life transition: Network changes, social skills and loneliness. In S. Duck & D. Perlman (Eds.), *The Sage series in personal relationships* (Vol. 1, pp. 193-217). London, England: Sage.

Waxman, L. D., & Reyes, L. M. (1987). *A status report of homeless families in America's cities—a 29-city survey.* Washington, DC: Conference of Mayors.

Zagacki, K. S., Honeycutt, J. M., & Edwards, R. (1992). The role of mental imagery and emotions in imagined interactions. *Communication Quarterly, 40,* 56-58.

14

CHEROKEE GENERATIVE METAPHORS

LISA R. PERRY

This chapter is a tentative first step in trying to unravel the generative metaphors that underlie the assumptions of the Cherokee worldview. A *generative metaphor* is one that underlies many other metaphors, a basic form of perception within a culture that is immediately recognizable and that can be used without explanation. For example, in English war is a generative metaphor, based on which we can *attack* a problem, *fight* cancer, *battle* disease, *conquer* a love. An analysis of the generative metaphor can give insight into the categories of a world hypothesis (Pepper, 1966).

It appears to be a characteristic of generative metaphors to play off of each other and to be interchangeable in terms of information conveyance. For example, in English *sports*, *sex*, and *war* as generative metaphors frequently overlap (Cohn, 1986; Perry, 1994). This may well be a trait of related generative metaphors. It should be of no surprise that Cherokee generative metaphors intertwine. Examining the metaphors can also reveal much about the role of women in the culture.

Cherokee generative metaphors appear to fall into at least three groups:[1] (a) *seed metaphors*, which are most often told using corn; (b) *balance metaphors*, which take the form of essential dualities; and (c) *weaving metaphors*, which often take the form of tapestry and baskets. Because the Cherokee do not view things as single, isolated acts but as processes, their generative metaphors reflect a worldview that is cyclical—focused on balance—and that promotes responsibility and equality. While the Western worldview is historically linear—following a line from the present into the future—the Cherokee view things in terms of cycles or loops; the past is integrally connected to the present and the future. Both the past and the present determine the future. The future is not viewed in terms of progress, implying constant "improvement," but in terms of pattern. Just as the past and present determine the future, the future will become the present and then the past that determines the future. To continue a productive cycle, one must be responsible in dealing with the present because the future does not spring into being with absolutely no connections to the past nor in turn with the next future. To the Cherokee, the future is not an abstract idea always waiting to happen, but a part of a cycle that does indeed reoccur.

SEED METAPHORS

In examining Cherokee stories, one of the first metaphors to come to light concerns seeds. It appears that one of the Cherokee generative metaphors is a seed-based metaphor. Aspects of the seed metaphors pervade the Cherokee worldview. Stories are viewed as seeds; they are planted in good soil and allowed to mature and bear fruit. Children, for example, are taught through stories. Children are not expected to understand the entire story all at once but to hold the story inside themselves; as they mature over time, the story will bear fruit for years, allowing the child to draw on this wisdom over a period of time. Of course, for seeds to grow the soil must be prepared. This is done by being an active member of a large and nurturing family and tribe from the moment one is born. The family and the tribe are the soil that feeds the children and allow them to grow. In turn, children become the soil in which the seeds of the history and the wisdom of the tribe are planted and from which a new crop will come. This sequence also exemplifies the cyclical nature of the Cherokee worldview.

---

[1]Personal communication from my grandmother. This is true of all Cherokee information in this chapter that is not otherwise credited.

In this method of raising children, responsibility becomes an integral part of a child's experience. Children learn how to behave in a culturally acceptable manner not because they will be dominated and punished by violence (e.g., hitting or beating), but because they have been taught to think through and recognize the long-term consequences of their actions, just as the seed sprouts and comes to offer its bounty to others. The Cherokee view is that responsibility begets responsibility and violence begets violence.

Another aspect of seed metaphors is how they promote a long-term view of events. By their nature, seeds promote patience, as does the raising of children. Seeds need to be planted and then given time to grow. Sowers plant their seeds and then wait, knowing that in time the corn will grow, mature, and bear fruit. It will not happen overnight; a crop must be carefully nurtured for a long time before it can be harvested. Lives built on such a metaphor lead to long- rather than short-term planning and thinking. Seeds must be taken care of; soil must be prepared and nurtured if good harvests are going to occur; the results of future harvests depend on what happened in past harvests. The Cherokee do not think they can dominate seeds and force them to grow. Seeds grow in their own time, affected by how they are handled. Growers, seeds, and the environment are joined in a cooperative effort, not a conflictive one.

The seed metaphor is most obvious in the Cherokee's special relationship with and to corn. Corn is viewed as a special gift to the Cherokee people. It is significant that in all of the stories the person who gives the gift of corn is always a woman. It is equally important that the corn women are often older. In fact, in all of the stories the corn woman is either a mother or a grandmother. "The Origin of Corn," reproduced in the Appendix, is an excellent example of this type of story. Also, the healer among the Cherokee is a Corn Woman.

BALANCE METAPHORS

A second set of metaphors that appear in the Cherokee worldview are the balance metaphors. The importance of maintaining ecological balance is the point of one of the most important stories that illustrates this metaphor. This story explains the Cherokee view of hunting and agriculture. Cherokee are not supposed to over hunt because it disturbs the balance and the results would be disastrous to all involved—humans and animals. In the Cherokee worldview, nature is to be treated with respect; cooperation and balance are the keys. Cherokee do not think of either hunting or agriculture as ways to dominate and control either animals or plants, as the following story illustrates. One of the major characters is Awi Usdi or Little Deer, chief of the deer (Awiakta, 1993). In Cherokee tradition, the corn and the deer are companions. Selu is the corn mother and her counterpart is Awi Usdi, teacher of the sacred law of respect to hunters and other people. Together, Selu and Awi Usdi represent the balance and harmony between female and male and between people and nature. The basic story of the Little Deer tales is that a very long time ago the hunters were killing and taking too many of the animals (evidently our problems in handling our environment are nothing new). Finally, the problem became so dire that the animals had to take some sort of action. They decided to have a meeting. In the meeting the animals discussed different solutions to their problem. Finally, Awi Usdi proposed a solution:

> "I see what we must do," he said.
> "We cannot stop the humans from hunting animals. That is the way it was meant to be. However, the humans are not doing things in the right way. If they do not respect us and hunt us only when there is real need, they may kill us all. I shall go now and tell the hunters what they must do. Whenever they wish to kill a deer, they must prepare in a ceremonial way. They must ask me for permission to kill one of us. Then, after they kill a deer, they must show respect to its spirit and ask for pardon. If the hunters do not do this, then I shall track them down. With my magic I will make their limbs crippled. Then they will no longer be able to walk or shoot a bow and arrow." Then Awi Usdi, Little Deer, did as he said. (Awiakta, 1993, p. 29)

This traditional story has many permutations, but in each the main point of this story remains. The law of respect and balance is sacred. It is eternal and immutable. One must take only with the utmost respect and one must give back with respect. Balance must be maintained. Selu and Awi Usdi, corn and deer, complement each other. Both are essential to keep balance, and both must be handled with respect. Both farming and hunting represent natural cycles. Balance extends beyond human and environment interaction to include the interaction between women and men. Each has a role to play. Both are needed to maintain balance, and are equally important. Balance metaphors do not promote singularity, domination, or hierarchy. Because the sexes are equally important and the female is not derived from the male, the female is an essential part of the culture. Both female and male carry the seeds needed to grow the next generation. Each supplies a vital component for life. This concept of balance does not promote hierarchy because, as anyone who has ever watched a scale balance realizes, balance requires equality among the elements involved.

Just as Western cultures' metaphors intertwine with each other, the Cherokee seed metaphors and balance metaphors intertwine. This intertwining cannot lead to derivational thinking.[2] Seeds and animals do not derive from humans. They stand with people and therefore deserve respect. The same is true of women and men. Women do not derive from men but both stand together as equals. Each contributes to the balance of life. Lives of all three—seeds, animals, and humans—intertwine, their cycles intersecting. All depend on each other and need mutual cooperation, respect, and nurturing for all to survive. Sex, for example, is coupled with life and cooperation.

One of the more striking examples of metaphors intertwining can be seen in the symbol of corn. Corn is considered to be one of the ultimate examples of balance and harmony of form and substance (Awiakta, 1993). Corn is born from union of the female and male flower, both of which, significantly, grow on the same plant. The female flowers grow on the corn stalk on a structure that will eventually become the ear. The male flowers grow higher up on the tassel and produce the corn's pollen. The female flowers, appearing as the silks, receive the pollen. After they receive the pollen, kernels start to grow and then fill with milk until they ripen and mature (Awiakta, 1993). This description of corn shows how both the seed metaphors and the balance metaphors help explain the world. The corn plant comes from seeds and bears seeds. But to become a bearer of seeds, a balance is needed. A balance of female and male is essential for the corn stalk to bear "fruit." To the Cherokee, the stalk of corn becomes a symbol or metaphor of the essential nature of gender balance.

The Cherokee view of women, then, is that of an equal and essential part of the world. This worldview is not singular and masculine but involves essential dualities including feminine and masculine. In fact, the feminine and the masculine are intertwined. This is illustrated by an incident that happened more than two centuries ago. A Cherokee chief, well known for his intelligence, shrewdness, and diplomacy, named Attakullakulla, had arrived to negotiate a treaty with the Whites. Members of his delegation included women, which when one remembers the stalk of corn, is the only way it could be: Women were (and had to be) an essential part of his delegation. These women were "as famous in war, and as powerful in council" as their male counterparts. Their presence also had a ceremonial significance: It showed honor for the other delegation. When Attakullakulla saw the White delegation his first response was, Where are your women? (Awiakta, 1993, pp. 92-93).

---

[2]See the introduction to this book for references and a discussion of derivational thinking.

The Cherokee were shocked to realize that the White delegation included no women. To the Whites, the absence of women was normal and natural. To the Cherokee, however, such a delegation had no balance and therefore no honor. Reverence for women/Mother Earth and for corn/life/spirit is interconnected such that disrespect for one signals disrespect for the others. To have no women in the delegation showed a marked disrespect for women and therefore a lack of balance. To the Cherokee this was a serious breech that called the intentions of the White men into question. They became wary of the Whites' motives, because to be so out of balance implied a very destructive mentality.

The further intertwining of metaphors can be seen in the Cherokee story of Awi Usdi and Selu. The cyclical worldview is long range. Corn must be handled with respect to achieve a good harvest year after year. The corn depends on humans and humans depend on corn. Balance. Wildlife must be handled with respect if there are going to be abundant supplies season after season. Again, wildlife depends on humans and humans depend on wildlife. All three—corn, wildlife, and humans—are intertwining threads in the cycle of life.

WEAVING METAPHORS

The intertwined elements of corn, human, and wildlife lead to the Cherokee generative metaphor of *weaving*. The Cherokee see things in terms of strands, webs, and connections. Weaving metaphors convey the importance of discerning patterns. They also convey the plurality and cyclical nature of life as the Cherokee see it. Singularity is not an underlying assumption, one cannot weave a tapestry with one thread, no basket can be made with only one reed. Weaving requires multiple strands or reeds, each important and having an integral part in the emerging pattern. These metaphors illuminate further the long-term way of viewing the world. Patterns evolve over time. They are made up of closely interconnecting parts. To see the entire pattern, past, present, and future have to be perceived.

Western hierarchy, like singularity, does not fit into the Cherokee weaving metaphor structure. To weave a pattern all of the parts are equally important. It even sounds odd to discuss one strand or reed as being more important than the others.

These metaphors often describe the complexity and interconnections of the world. A good example of this type of metaphor concerns baskets. One of the most common baskets is the *doublewoven basket*, also known as the Cherokee basket (Awiakta, 1993). The doublewoven basket has two patterns interwoven together. One pattern forms the outside of the basket and the other pattern forms the inside. Often, this basket is used as a metaphor to describe the relationship between Selu and the people. The outer pattern is considered a path to Selu. The inner pattern represents Selu herself. Therefore, the path is walked together, balanced, and connected.

The weaving metaphors expose a worldview that sees life as connected in terms of relationships and groups. No individual stands alone, as in Western worldview, but is a part of a tapestry or web of relationships involving both humans and nature. Humans do not, cannot, stand outside of nature because they are so completely tied to the natural world. The Western worldview of science and objectivity make no sense in the Cherokee worldview.

CONCLUSION

The Cherokee made an illuminating connection between the way the Europeans treated corn and how they in turn treated other people. The Europeans took corn from the New World, treating it as nothing more than a food grain, divesting it of any teaching and spiritual value. Eventually, corn became equated with peasants; it became "peasant" food (Awiakta, 1993). Awiakta pointed out that Europeans usually link corn to the expendable, including both animals and people, leading to sayings such as "Corn is for livestock or peasants" (p. 223). She believes that linking corn and people reveals the European view that indigenous people were expendable. The European system and worldview allowed them to classify certain groups of people with animals and therefore render them expendable. This linkage allowed the Cherokee to gage the European's view of life. How the Europeans treated corn was a good indication of their respect for life in general. To use and consume without thought for the long-term consequences was obviously the European way.

> Columbus took the grain-only and ate it. . . . To use and consume was his cultural habit. . . . Thus Columbus sounded the keynote of the attitude of Manifest Destiny: that the powerful of Europe, being superior, had the right to "use and consume" not only the new land but also its indigenous people, who were "uncivilized" and "pagan," that is, expendable. Within a century, the Native peoples of the Caribbean—some estimates say five to seven million—were dead. (Awiakta, 1993, pp. 222-223)

The weaving metaphor weaves the others. Seed stories are planted in the mind and as they mature, story and life interweave. Lives of female and male, people and animals, all weave around each other, twined together, to achieve balance. Because all of life is intertwined and interrelated, respect is very important and the idea of respect is woven into the stories.

The Cherokee worldview, as ascertained from an analysis of these metaphors, is shaped by seeing things in terms of intertwining cycles, balances, and long-range terms. This is in direct opposition to the Western worldview, which is linear and hierarchical, involving domination, conquering, and short-range thinking. After examining these metaphor systems it becomes very clear that when White Europeans, mostly men, came into contact with the Cherokee, two completely different worlds collided. The Europeans' derivational thinking led them to dismiss the women of the Cherokee people, and to misjudge the men.

The Cherokee metaphors unveil a worldview emphasizing balance, respect, equality, and responsibility. Identity is defined by group membership and each individual is responsible to the group. Instead of hierarchy, lives intertwine together each with its own contribution. These metaphors generate a worldview that is based on balance and responsibility, and concerned with cycles and long-range planning.

APPENDIX: THE ORIGIN OF CORN

At one time there was a very old woman who had two grandsons. These two grandsons were always hunting. They hunted deer and wild turkeys. They always had plenty to eat.

Later on, after many hunting trips, when they got ready to go hunting early in the morning, they were cleaning their guns. When their grandmother noticed that they were ready to go, she thought to herself, "They are getting ready to go hunting," so she went to them where they were cleaning their guns, outside the fenced-in yard.

When the grandmother came to them they were busily cleaning their guns. She said to them, "I see that you are getting ready to go hunting," and they replied, "Yes. We are going to hunt deer today."

"Well, when you come back, I'll have the most delicious of dinners ready. I'm going to cook all of the old meat, and I'm going to put into it something they call corn and we're going to drink the broth from it," she said to the young men.

"All right," said the young men.

When they got to the forest they wondered about the word corn that she had used. They did not know what that was, and they wondered where she got it.

"I wonder where corn comes from?" they asked each other. "When we get home, we'll find out," they said. They killed a deer, shouldered it and went home.

When they got home, they saw the large pot bubbling. They noticed that with the meat, corn in small ground-up pieces was boiling in there. (If anyone had ever seen it before, he would have known what it was; but then these boys had never seen it before.)

They asked their grandmother, "What is that that you have in the pot?"

"It is called grits."

They didn't ask her where she got it.

When they ate their dinner, the young men had the most delicious meal that they had ever had. After dinner they told their grandmother what a superb meal she had cooked. The grandmother was pleased.

"Well, tomorrow at noon we will have some more delicious food."

The next day they went hunting again, but they already had some dried turkeys. So the grandmother cooked these dried turkeys and cooked grits with them.

When they returned home that evening with their bag of turkeys, dinner was announced. With this meat were these grits, and the young men said, "This is the best meal that we have ever had." They thanked their grandmother again and told her that her food was delicious.

The grandmother was very pleased and said, "I'm so happy that you said what you did."

Next day they again went to the forest. While they were in the forest, one of them keep thinking about the corn. "This thing she calls corn . . . she said that today about noon she is going to starting cooking again," said one to the other; and the other said, "Yes, that's what she said."

"I'll go hide around somewhere and see where she gets it if you want me to," said one.

"All right," said the other. "You had better go before she begins cooking."

So one of them went. This thing called corn was troubling this young man; so he hid behind the smokehouse and watched for his grandmother.

Later on the grandmother came carrying a large pan and went into the smokehouse. The young man peeped through a small hole. When the grandmother got into the smokehouse, she put the pan under where she was standing. Then she stuck both of her sides, and when she hit her sides grits fell from every part of her body. They fell until the pan became full. When she came out of the smokehouse, she carried this pan of grits, dumped them into the pot, and began cooking them.

That's what the young man learned, and he went back to his brother and told him about it. When he arrived where his brother was, his brother asked him what he had learned.

He said to his brother, "This delicious food of Grandmother's that we have been eating comes from her body. She shakes it off from all over her body. She puts a pan under her. She strikes her sides, and it falls off her body and falls into the pan until it is full, and that is what we have been eating," he told his brother.

His brother said, "We really eat an unsavory thing, don't we!" So they decided that they would not eat any more of it when they got home.

When they arrived home, their grandmother had dinner ready. Again she had the same kind of food. They both didn't each much.

"What's wrong? You're not eating very much. Don't you like me?" said their grandmother.

The young men said, "No. We're just too tired from walking so much in our hunting."

"But I think that you don't like me," she said. "Or maybe you learned something somewhere, and that's the reason that you don't want to eat," they were told.

At that moment the grandmother became ill. She knew that they had found out [her secret]. The grandmother took to bed, and she began to talk to them about what they should do.

"Now that I'm in bed, I'm going to die." (She told them all about what was going to happen in the future.) "When you bury me, you must put a large fence around me and bury me just right out there. Something will grow from right in the middle of my grave. This thing will grow up to be tall. It will flower at the top, and in the lower part will come out beautiful tassels, and inside of them will be kernels. It will bear two or three ears of corn with corn silk on them."

"You must leave the ears alone and take care of the plant. Put a fence around it. They [the ears] will dry; they will be very white; the shuck will be brown and crisp; and the silk will be dark brown. That is when you gather it."

"This thing they call corn is I. This corn will have its origin in me."

"You must take the kernels off the cob and plant them. Store them away until spring. When spring comes, make spaced-out holes in the ground and put about two of the kernels in each hole. By doing this you will increase your supply—and it is surpassing good food—and when it sprouts, it will go through the various stages of growth that you will have seen in this one of mine."

"Then it will bear corn that you can use, either to boil (boiled corn is very good to eat all summer long, while it is green) or in winter you can use it to make meal."

"I will be the Corn-Mother," said the old woman (a long time ago, they said).

That's the injunction that the young men were taught to carry out. They thought about this deeply as they were burying her after she died. After they buried her, they made the fence; and all that summer [the corn plant] grew and bore corn just as she told them it would do, and when the corn became dry, they gathered it and took the kernels off the cobs.

Then again next spring they planted it. Then the two young men said, "It would be better if we each had a wife."

One of the young men said, "Let's just one of us get a wife. You get a wife, and I'll be a bachelor and live with you."

The other said, "All right," and left to search for a wife.
The young man said to the one who left to get a wife, "Just walk some distance over there, blow into your hands, and there will be a girl run to you."

So he arrived away off into the forest near a house, I believe. In that house was an old couple with a large number of young women.

These young women were all outside playing. Some of these young women were frolicking about, and others were laughing and making a lot of noise.

The young man came quite near, blew into his hands, and whistled. One of the young women who was playing stopped and said, "I'm going to stop playing because someone is whistling for me," and left the group. She ran directly to the young man. The young man said to her, "We'll marry, if it's all right with you."

She said, "All right." So they went to his home.

The young man told her that in the spring they would plant corn, and each year they would plant more and more of it. So when spring came, they used their hoes to make holes so they could plant corn. They hoed and hoed and had a very large field of corn, and that was the beginning of there being so much corn. And they remembered what the old woman had said to them, "I will be the Corn-Mother," she had said. "Don't ever forget where I am buried," she had told them when she talked to them.

From this beginning there became so much corn that everyone in the world had some. They say that corn had its beginning from a human being, that the plant called corn started from a woman, and that when this man took a wife, they had such a huge field that they had much corn and much food to eat.

That's what I know, and that's the end of it: that's all.(Awiakta, 1993, pp. 10-14)

REFERENCES

Awiakta, M. (1993). *Selu: Seeking the corn-mother's wisdom*. Golden, CO: Fulcrum.

Cohn, C. (1986). Sex and death in the rational world of defense intellectuals. *Signs, 12*, 687-718.

Pepper, S. C. (1966). *Concept and quality: A world hypothesis*. La Salle, IL: Open Court.

Perry, L. R. (1994). *Derivational thinking*. Unpublished manuscript, University of Florida at Gainesville.

15

SEXUAL HARASSMENT AND CAT CALLS IN THE BLACK COMMUNITY

LaTASHA LaJOURN FARMER

In spring 1994, I enrolled in a course that dealt with metaphor and derivational thinking. One of the assignments was to watch a video of a Phil Donahue talk show on cat calls. We were to ask three women and three men about their views on cat calls. One repeated response I received was that "women do [cat calls] too." The responses and my own perception differed from that of my classmates who thought such behavior restricted to men. These differences led my professor and me to look at the idea of verbal interplay. Verbal interplay or word games involve two-party flirting. I began to explore the idea that members of the Black community may use a definition of sexual harassment at least within that community that differs from how harassment is defined by the White community. The responses I received sparked the beginnings of this chapter.

This chapter is a preliminary study of a matter that needs to be studied more extensively. Since I first wrote this chapter, I have seen further behavior supporting my hypothesis. I cannot, of course, present this chapter as a homogenous representation of the Black community. Verbal interplay can be influenced by age, class, and geographical area. Yet, were we to deny the possibility of cultural differences regarding sexual harassment, we may be in danger of placing cultural restraints on the Black community. Verbal interplay is not exclusive to the Black community but its existence may indicate one problem presented by current definitions of sexual harassment.

A male friend was interested in a young woman in one of his classes. He wanted to approach her but he overheard a conversation between White students about sexual harassment and decided against talking to her. He was afraid that he would be accused of harassment. Later, the woman approached him and he discovered that she also had been interested. Because of situations such as the one just cited, sexual harassment needs to be redefined. Verbal interplay, as a mode of communication, needs to be explored before members of the Black community begin to feel uncomfortable with flirting. The responses from my peers were all in a similar vein, so I combined them in a collective voice.

Sexual harassment as defined by the Equal Employment Opportunity Commission (EEOC), the Executive Office of the President, and the majority of universities is "unwelcome sexual advances, requests for sexual favors, and other verbal or physical conduct of a sexual nature that is unsolicited." Sexual harassment can be initiated by either a person in authority or a peer. Sexual harassment is not limited to the workplace nor does it require sexual favors. Victims can also include a person who is affected by the harassment of someone else.

The women and men I interviewed gave definitions that paralleled but also diverged from that of the EEOC. Initially, sexual harassment was defined as any touching or rubbing. The definition was broadened to include badgering, name calling, verbal filth, involvement of blackmail or bribery and violating the boundaries the other party has set. My respondents considered hissing or cat calls such as "Yo, baby! Hey, baby!" to be signs of rudeness more than harassment. The important fact about this definition is that unsolicited sexual advances are not considered harassment. Only when those advances "get out of hand" (i.e., because of badgering or name calling), do they turn into harassment.

Certain key points signify the line dividing verbal interplay and sexual harassment. Verbal interplay is not offensive because both parties are engaged. Even if the attention is unsolicited, the recipient has the choice to ignore the advance or continue the flirting game and it ends if not reciprocated. In verbal interplay, one party initiates a verbal move while the other responds with an equal verbal response. Neither party dominates and both understand that the game can end at any time. A woman or man can initiate the verbal game and both parties have free choice of participation. Verbal interplay is a way for two parties to learn more about each other and to discover boundaries.

I was given several examples of flirting instigated by women and men and have included some here.

Male: "Hey baby. You look good."
Female: "Oh no, baby. It's all about you. You look damn good."

Female or Male: "I'm just a squirrel trying to get a nut in your world."

Female: "I know you want me. I saw you looking at [eyeing] me."
Male: "Yeah, man. You caught me." [I'm busted. You found me out].

Male: "You want me, don't you?"
Female: "How you found out?"

Female: "Every time I turn around I keep seeing you. You following me, ain't you?"
Male: "Nah, you following me."

Male: "Hey, baby. Com'ere."
Female: "Why can't you come to me?"

Female: "Let me go get my car and then I'll come back and give you my number."
Male: "No, you might not come back. I need to get a number now."
Female: "I'll come back."
Male: "Look, you can give me a fake number, you can give an 800 number. Just so I got something to show."
Female: "All right, 1-800 . . ."
[Laugher and then conversation resumes.]
Second male: "What number were you about to give?"
Female: "The number for MCI."

Verbal interplay can occur between friends, lovers or strangers. Sometimes, language can be sexually explicit; other times it is simply suggestive. A major component is a relaxed environment. Hostility can turn a verbal game into a verbal attack. Each individual has set boundaries on what is and is not appropriate. In a verbal game, those boundaries are not to be crossed under any circumstances and if they are, the game ends. For a verbal game to be successful, both women and men have to be on equal footing. Even if one party initiates, both parties have the chance to continue, monopolize, or change the game. Two interviewees offered an example from Zora Neal Hurston's *Their Eyes Were Watching God*. In chapter 10, Janey finally meets Tea Cake. He flirts with her, which Janey calls "play." After they have talked and flirted a bit, Janey realizes that she still does not know his name. When she asks, his response is as follows:

> ". . . De name mah mama gimme is Vergible Woods. Dey calls me Tea Cake for short."
> "Tea Cake! So you sweet as all dat?" She laughed and he gave her a little cut-eye look to get her meaning.
> "Ah may be guilty. You better try me and see." (p. 93)

The fact that Tea Cake is willing to "play" with Janey, not only in a game of chess but verbally, gives Janey a sense of freedom. Tea Cake, who comes to Janey as an equal, offers the kind of relationship she did not experience in her first two marriages. The example of Janey and Tea Cake illustrates the concept of verbal interplay described in my interviews. For Janey, the strongest effect of the verbal game with Tea Cake was how she felt. Playing the game was fun and sensual. Janey was able to explore her sexuality in a way that her previous marriages had suppressed. Her former husbands sought to control any sexual expression, but Tea Cake, in flirting with her, created a space for her sexual freedom.

Verbal interplay, as exhibited by members of the black community is also a space for sexual freedom. Women and men are able to explore their sexuality, create boundaries, and learn the boundaries of the opposite sex. Verbal interplay can be harmless flirting but it can also lead to a relationship. As I stated before, verbal games are not universal to the Black community. Several interviewees explored environment as an influence on types of verbal interplay. Within some areas of the Black community and among certain members, cat calls such as "Hey, baby" are acceptable. At the same time, some women and men would find this behavior offensive. One woman suggested that verbal interplay would be more prevalent on college campuses than in high school because of a more relaxed environment.

Two cases often discussed in response to my questions were the Anita Hill-Clarence Thomas confrontation and the Mike Tyson rape trial. In the Hill harassment case, the biggest issue raised was the time factor. No one offered an opinion as to what the decision should have been, but many questioned why she had let so much time pass. One young woman suggested that Hill and Thomas' level in the community and Thomas' nomination to a high position may have influenced the eventual charges. Part of verbal interplay is the ability of both parties to choose to participate. If Hill found Thomas' advances inappropriate, why did she let them continue? The participants in this study were not interested in placing blame on Hill, but in understanding her choice to condone an unwanted behavior by keeping silent. One explanation offered was that Thomas may have taken a culturally sanctioned act into an area that was deemed inappropriate. Hill may have felt powerless to stop Thomas' advances. Yet, there were still questions. The women whom I interviewed did not believe in accepting unwanted behavior for any reason and the men had witnessed ways in which women could fend for themselves.

Discussing the Hill case seemed to be an important part of finding a definition of sexual harassment, as was the Mike Tyson trial. Although Tyson was accused of rape, the trial elicited some widely varying conceptions of sexual harassment. Among my acquaintances, the alleged victim received more criticism than did Tyson and understanding why involves verbal interplay. Most young Black women understand that after a certain time of night, men consider visits to be "booty calls." The time can fluctuate but after 11 and definitely after midnight, a woman who makes a late night visit is considered to be condoning any sexual activity that may occur. "Booty call" time is understood and if a woman does not wish to engage in sex then she does not visit. A couple of young men summed up "booty call" time perfectly. One was approached by a young woman at a party about 2 in the morning. He invited her to visit but told her, "It's 2:30 and ain't nothin' open but legs." Both women and men who participated in my interviews believed that the young woman who accused Tyson of rape should have known better especially because everyone knows "what's up at that time of night."

Verbal interplay can be natural communication among individuals in some groups. My respondents represented verbal interplay, a serious but light hearted game, as an instance of a Black woman's ability to take things less personally than White women. Unanimous among the interviewees was the belief that White women take everything too seriously. My participants discussed the differences between the relationships of Black women and men and those of White women and men. The possibility and the nature of verbal interplay seemed to lie in the fact that Black women and men were more equal than their White counterparts. Important to verbal interplay is equal distribution of power that was believed to be more possible in the Black community.

One woman stated that White women looking from the outside tended to find and draw parallels between Black and White relationships. White women were said to classify black relationships according to White standards. Each interviewee talked of the parallels between Black and White relationships but the black relationship was established as a separate entity. Black women, who could better hold onto and express power, could initiate and participate in verbal games without being dominated. If domination became a factor, they could end the game.

One woman talked about her job and the fact that the White men will not flirt with the White women but they will flirt with her. She leaves them notes or touches them on the bottom but they do not touch her back. Her explanation was that they were too afraid. She does not touch Black men because they will touch back. Black men are quicker to flirt and initiate verbal interplay.

All these factors do not mean the absence of sexual harassment in the Black community. My Black women respondents, however, believe themselves to be better equipped to handle harassing situations. Redefining sexual harassment is a necessary part of maintaining a cultural norm in the Black community. A redefinition would also enable Black youth to continue verbal games without the threat of legal ramifications, which I believe is important. Culturally sanctioned by members of the Black community, verbal word games permit both Black women and men to explore sexual freedom.

16

THE STIFLING OF WOMEN'S VOICES: MEN'S MESSAGES FROM MEN'S MOVEMENT BOOKS

DAVID NATHARIUS

In 1991, Susan Faludi wrote in *Backlash*:

> Feminism's agenda is basic: It asks that women not be forced to "choose" between public justice and private happiness. It asks that women be free to define themselves—instead of having their identity defined for them, time and again, by their culture and by their men. (xxiii)

Faludi's subtitle was: *The Undeclared War Against American Women*. In 1995, it appears that this "war against American women" was no longer undeclared. From the Anita Hill-Clarence Thomas sexual harassment hearings to the O.J. Simpson trial and its fall out of spousal abuse to the "angry White men" rebellion represented by attacks on abortion rights and affirmative action, a plethora of evidence demonstrated a threat to the social and economic gains made by women since the mid-1970s (Tavris, 1992). Most evident was that the political system on which many feminists relied to respond to the serious messages of women's movements responds as well to counter messages that diminish or discount women's rights issues.

Attacks on affirmative action mounted by Governor Pete Wilson in California appeared to ignore the simple fact that White men, who represent only one third of the nation's population, comprise almost 90% of the senior managers and professionals and, of the country's 400 wealthiest persons, 368 are White males (Chappell, 1995). And, although women are reaching parity in medical and legal schools, they are not making gains as "politicians, lawmakers, policymakers, world leaders" (Goodman, 1995, p. B9). Reardon (1995) pointed out that "of the total number of managerial/professional employees, 44 per cent are women. Yet study after study reports that in large companies less than 5 per cent of senior managers are women" (p. 3). In fact, the 1994 national election diminished the gains that women legislators had achieved in the 1992 vote. It seems clear that the backlash was real as the 1996 national and many local elections demonstrated.

Nowhere is the backlash against women's gains more evident than in several popular books that argue the poor state of the U.S. male (e. g . Greenstein, 1993; Kimbrell, 1995; Kimmel & Messner, 1992). These books present messages that men have not been better off than women, and that, in fact, men may be worse off in several different categories. The general theme revolves around the argument that men are actually the victims of social pressures requiring them to perform in ways not conducive to mental or physical health. This basic argument developed in the mid-1970s as male authors attempted to combat the growing awareness about women's issues. In the late 1990s, the arguments of the "oppressed male" seem to have taken center court for many men and have apparently diminished the willingness of many men (and women) to listen to and understand the women's voices that remind us that we are not making much progress. In reviewing the 1995 National Governors Association meeting, Barbara Yost (1995) commented:

> Two years after the Year of the Woman, New Jersey's Whitman is the only female governor in America. . . . So it was left to a bunch of men to debate the future of welfare, an issue that involves mostly women. . . . And it was left to a bunch of white men and one white woman to debate affirmative action. (p. B7)

Clearly, many people no longer listen to women's voices, which have been replaced by messages that men (mostly White) are victims and need to become aware of how to improve their own opportunities to make choices.

In this chapter, I examine the developing perception of men as victims rather than oppressors. This perception results in an attitude of "getting back" at women rather than attempting to understand women's personal, professional, and political issues with men. Such attitudes ignore many concerns of women and, consequently, discount, diminish, and trivialize women's voices. Specific reflection of this masculine reaction can be seen by examining three books that have become major expressions of how men react to women's perspectives. The three books are, *The Hazards of Being Male* (Goldberg, 1987), *Fire in the Belly* (Keen, 1991), and *The Myth of Male Power* (Farrell, 1993). These books argue that men actually are the victims in their social and professional relationships with women rather than the oppressors or controllers as feminists have long claimed. Not incidentally the messages of these three books continue to be dominant themes of more recent books about the male condition (Cose, 1995; Kimbrell, 1995; Thomas, 1993).

First, it is appropriate to review what the majority of women's voices are saying. They ask that men understand the need for moving toward gender equality in all contexts: socially, politically, professionally, and personally. Furthermore, they ask that men (and women) develop ways of integrating what is essentially White male bases of power into a more balanced system of exerting and responding to influence and control. Women seek the same freedom of choices as men and request (in some cases, demand) that men recognize and value the perceptions and perspectives of women as equally as they value perceptions and perspectives of other men (e.g., Goodman, 1991; Hagan, 1992; Reardon, 1995; Renzetti & Curran, 1993).

As the following books are reviewed it becomes clear that the authors have little interest in fully understanding the messages from women. Rather, their responses either disregard or diminish the feminists concerns.

In 1976, Goldberg's *The Hazards of Being Male* became a widely read and quoted source for men attempting to understand how they were being affected by the women's liberation movement. The book offers information to men that suggests that men are not necessarily better off than women just because they are men. This documentation includes the evidence that men have shorter life spans than women, are more susceptible to most forms of cancer, have higher rates of vascular and heart problems, have a significantly larger percentage of alcohol and drug problems, and in general are much worse off than women physically, spiritually, and emotionally. This book, currently in its "Anniversary Edition" (Goldberg, 1987), still has a major readership. The newer edition does not appear to have updated any of its research sources, most of which are from the early 1970s and earlier. More importantly, for this chapter, Goldberg did not really address the primary issues with which the modern feminist movement has been concerned: social and professional equity. In his last chapter, essentially an epilogue, titled "Out of the Harness: The Free Male," Goldberg developed a credo for the liberated male:

> The free male will constantly reaffirm his right and need to develop and to grow, to be total and fluid and to have no less than a state of total well being. He will celebrate all of the many dimensions of himself, his strength and his weakness, his achievements and his failures, his sensuality, his affectionate and loyal responses to women and men. He will follow his own personal growth path. (p. 184)

This statement reflects a concern for the limitations placed on men by society and culture. However, what is most disturbing about the statement is that it is ultimately drawn after several chapters of explaining what women have that men do not or how women are a major cause for the limitations of men. In chapters such as "The Lost Art of Buddyship," Goldberg (1987) deplored the absence of male friendships, while "Marriage: Guilt by Association" suggests that marriage and responsibility severely limit the free, spontaneous impulses that men have naturally. In describing an event in which a husband is arrested for wife beating, Goldberg characterized it as a "telescoped version of what so often happens to the once autonomous, impulsive male when he begins to adjust his rhythm to the needs of his wife" (p. 145). Suggesting that marriage causes men to give up "pleasurable and important" things, Goldberg said they react like little boys who think they have been caught doing something wrong. Such a man turns his wife into a permission-giver and denies his own identity because he sees patterns and interests as being unworthy or selfish.

The disturbing element here is the impression that a relationship with a woman caused these effects on men. Consequently, the image of man as suppressed and limited by woman emerges as a believable myth. More insidiously, it also implies that the "free male" must not allow women to exert control over his life. The issue of equality is not acknowledged or addressed. Men who may believe these assertions would certainly not be motivated to be more open and responsive to developing mutual respect for women in their interpersonal transactions.

Fifteen years after the first appearance of *The Hazards of Being Male*, two new books emerged that argue that the reasons for the poverty of male spiritual and emotional health initially addressed by Goldberg and others center around the failure by men to understand their archetypal tribal origins. *Fire in the Belly* by Keen (1991), along with

Bly's *Iron John* (1990), reflect the foundations for a men's movement focused on inner self-discovery through "tribal" contact with other men. These books either spawned or tapped into the new men's movement, generally identified as the mythopoetic movement, and shifted the emphasis from developing ways of coping with the ambiguity of new social roles created by the feminist movement (as did Goldberg's book) to an emphasis on discovering the elements in men that make them uniquely masculine. The most publicized and often satirized process for this discovery is the "wild man weekend," in which men from various social backgrounds gather for an intensive group interaction usually as a camp or tribal experience. Elements of these gatherings include chanting, singing, dancing, sweat lodges with or without clothes, drumming, and sometimes intensive one on one encounters with each other and/or with the camp facilitators (Brod, 1992).

Keen's (1991) book can be characterized as the search for the uniqueness of the male spirit. In Keen's terms, the book is an invitation to a quest for finding, not the "real" man, but the "whole man." His major argument is that men have been unconsciously influenced by the cultural power of women and, for men to become more complete and to understand the dimensions of influence that have controlled their lives, they must separate themselves from the influence of women. In his introductory chapter, Keen stated: "I would guess that a majority of men never break free, never define manhood by weighing and testing their own experience. And the single largest reason is that we never acknowledge the primal power WOMAN wields over us" (p. 14).

Keen (1991) certainly expressed an understanding of what women want when he stated: "First and foremost, women want what they have been denied—justice, equality, respect, and power" (p. 5). He proceeded, however, to make a claim similar to Goldberg, that women have been the reason for men's inability to function fully as human beings. Actually, Keen's assertion is that it is WOMAN (in upper case letters) that has caused the problem. In other words, it is the *myth* of woman that is embedded in men's unconscious.

> It is the WOMAN in our heads, more than the women in our beds or boardrooms who cause most of our problems. . . . So long as our house is haunted by the ghost of WOMAN we can never live gracefully with any woman. If we continue to deny that she lives in the shadows she will continue to have power over us. (p. 6)

Keen then suggested that men must make a journey that takes them away from women, into the world of men, before they can return to "the everyday world to love an ordinary woman" (p. 18). What Keen described as the world of men appears to be the unconscious psyche that men have never explored sufficiently to break through the social and cultural demands placed on "manhood." Keen devoted a large segment of the book to exploring the mythical, archetypal elements that have kept men from fully exploring and understanding themselves as men.

So, the journey that Keen wants man, or men, to take, is an exploration of all that is missing from his rational, responsible life. He wants men to explore those dimensions of their lives that he claims have been suppressed or, in some cases, lost from the male awareness: the playboy, the *puer aeternis*, Peter Pan. Additionally, he seemed quite clear that the only way to accomplish this journey is by men removing themselves from women, and exploring these dimensions with men—in groups, in dialogues with male friends, in extensive periods of interaction as well as in isolation and alone, in reflection and introspection. For Keen, "Man" is a significantly different creature from "Woman" and, therefore, must discover his manness through explorations with other men. Also clear is that Keen does not suggest that men examine themselves through external parameters. Throughout Keen's book is a continuing use of oxymorons, among them: peaceful virility, and fierce gentleman. This may be Keen's way of alerting men to the difficult task they face as men to keep their strength but only to exert it in positive directions, in committing themselves to just causes: the preservation of the earth, the importance of family, honest and socially committed forms of government and commerce. Perhaps the tension of these contradictory terms serves to remind that the journey that men must take is not easy and that only a few men will be willing to experience it.

Keen's (1991) last section is: "Men and Women: Coming Together;" interesting terminology after spending much previous time alluding to the sexual emphasis that so often permeates men's thinking, usually in a negative way. Could he not have used "Joining Together," or "Becoming Together?" Here he attends to the processes of men connecting with women in ways that do not carry the old mythic stereotypes of feminine and masculine. Keen even suggested the abandonment of those terms: "In my judgment, we would gain much clarity if we ceased using the words "masculine" and "feminine" except to refer to the stereotypes of the genders that have been historically predominant" (p. 214). He wants to "remain with the real mystery of man and woman [rather] than the false mystification of the masculine and feminine. As nearly as I can tell, I, being a man, have nothing feminine about me" (p. 214).

If men accept that last statement, then it is clear their communication with women will probably be maintained at a level of disregard for even attempting to understand women's perspectives in any relational interaction. Moreover, it totally ignores what all of the recent gender research suggests—that men and women are much more similar than different (Wood, 1994).

Although *The Hazards of Being Male* (Goldberg, 1987) and *Fire in the Belly* (Keen, 1991) represent different attempts at male enlightenment, neither appears to address ways in which men can develop a supportive and enlightened sensitivity to some fundamental women's issues. Goldberg had little to say about how men can support and understand women's issues. Keen implied that this support and understanding will come about as a natural result of men freeing themselves from the limitations that have been placed on them through unconscious myths. What emerges is an implicit conclusion that talking with women will not really help men in resolving their own issues, and, men have little concern for women' s issues.

An examination of the third book in this review, *The Myth of Male Power* (Farrell, 1993), reveals some fundamental reasoning that perpetuates a distancing from integrating the masculine and feminine perspectives of "getting it." Farrell, a self-described feminist who has become a "masculist," suggested a definition of power as "having control over one's own life" (p. 48). Working from this definition, Farrell proceeded to argue that men have very little control over their own lives and the primary reason is, of course, women. In Farrell's perspective, men have actually become victims of the cultural and social influences that require men to be protectors, providers, and guardians of women (and children). In chapter one, reflecting Goldberg's perspective of almost two decades earlier, Farrell listed several areas in which this male powerlessness is manifested: shorter life expectancy than women, higher suicide rate, more likely to be victims of violence, more money spent on women than men. Additionally, he pointed out that men are expected to be the primary wage earners, to pay the major household expenses such as mortgages, and to provide the major support for children in the household. To provide a foundation for understanding how men are not in control of their lives, Farrell used the "Women as Nigger" analogy: "But what none of us realized was how each sex was the other's slave in different ways. . . . The comparison is useful because it is not until we understand how men were also women's servants that we get a clear picture of the sexual *division* of labor" (p. 39). Within this framing, Farrell developed his arguments that men have actually never been better off than women and, in fact, since the women's movement, men have lost even more power in their social and professional existence.

In examining the advances that women have made since the 1970s, Farrell (1993) offered several areas in which women have significantly greater power over their own lives than men have over men's lives. He developed the "emergence of the multi-option woman and the no-option man" (p. 52). He compared the options that modern woman has: "work full time, mother full time, some combination of working and mothering" with the options that modern man has: "work full time, work full time, work full time" (pp. 52-53). Farrell argued that women have maintained greater power over their lives than men because men have always been more disposable. Men have been expected to fight the wars, pull the plows and carts, and defend women from attack and violence. Some analogies offered include: "Gladiators and Their Virgins" (p. 75), "Christ and His Nuns" (p. 88), football players and cheerleaders (pp. 75, 76, 167ff). He argued that men are more violent than women because "the deeper purpose of violence against men was to prevent violence against women" (p. 75).

Farrell (1993) developed the metaphor of the "Glass Cellars" to present the negative aspects of the working male: evidence supporting the assertion that men are the overwhelming victims of occupational death—94% and that the most hazardous occupations are almost totally male (97%-98%), compared to the safe occupations that are almost totally female (97%-99%). He extended the argument by demonstrating that, although women may receive lower pay than men, they are largely in jobs that have much more flexibility in hours, safer environments, and lower psychological risks. He also explored the unequal obligation that most men face in serving in the armed services. Women in the armed forces will continue to have the "choice to: 1. Enter combat, 2. Not enter combat" (p. 127). And, historically, men have been the overwhelming victims of death and injury due to warfare. He probed why the incidence of young male suicide rates has increased, whereas young women's decreased; explored the increased differential between life spans of women and men; reviewed the pressures placed on males in executive and professional positions; examined the phenomenon of violence; and concluded that males are much more likely to be victims of violent crime than women. He suggested that male violence is a result of the *powerless* feeling that men have. Violence is "but a minute's worth of superficial power to compensate for years of underlying powerlessness," which is why he said it is committed disproportionately by Blacks and men (p. 125). One has to wonder if he really meant to distinguish Blacks from men, and what it suggests about the movement he promoted that he made such a claim, even if he did so "unconsciously." He suggested "If we really want men to commit crime as infrequently as women, we can start by not expecting men to provide for women more than we expect women to provide for men" (p. 216).

Finally, Farrell (1993) examined the area he argued is ultimately the most favorable toward women, the role government has taken in developing protections for women's rights. He reviewed how women charged with the same crimes as men are more likely to receive lighter sentences or even be freed on probation or to a counselor. He explained that even in cases of homicide, the defenses strongly favor women defendants:

> Neither men nor women are exempt from killing loved ones. The difference is in what happens to them when they do. Twelve distinct female-only defenses allow a woman who commits a premeditated murder to have the charges dropped or significantly reduced. No man has successfully used any of these defenses in similar circumstances. Nor do men have any equivalent "male-only" defenses. (p. 254)

In discussing "The Politics of Sex," Farrell developed the argument that sexual harassment is primarily a female power base in which males are powerless. He claimed that sexual harassment legislation in its present form makes all men unequal to all women. Exploring the unequal power thus given women in the workplace, Farrell cited the examples of Anita Hill and Dr. Frances Conley at Stanford University. In both cases, these accusations made major news headlines and both women were hailed as heroines by a large portion of the population—at least of the female population. What was not examined thoroughly, according to Farrell, was the background of the women who made the charges. He objected to making "judgments about men as sexual harassers without knowing that the women making the accusations were possibly bitter about promotions" (p. 306).

In "The Politics of Rape," Farrell (1993) examined the issues surrounding rape as an act of sex or violence, questioned to what degree "date rape" is actually a crime, and the degree the woman is responsible for the act of rape. He argued that "If we want to stop date rape by men, we have to also stop 'date passivity' by women. Thus far, women *retain* the old option to be passive and take indirect initiatives" (p. 313). He seemed to be suggesting that the act of rape, at least date rape, is an act for which a woman must take as much responsibility as the man. He also assessed the research on false accusations of rape, citing one study that has "thoroughly" studied rape accusations and concluded that "A total of 60 percent of the original rape allegations were false" (p. 322). Were this particular chapter to be believed, the result could be little besides paranoia on the part of men regarding how their lives could be ruined forever if they even put themselves in an interpersonal situation where the women could cry rape, usually in spurious allegations.

Clearly, *The Myth of Male Power* (Farrell, 1993) shares with Keen (1991) and Goldberg (1987) the claim that men have really been the more powerless of the genders. Farrell couched his assertion in the form of a response to all of the gains accomplished by women since the 1970s and specifically as an argument against many of the claims of "the feminists."

However, in using the term, *the feminists*, Farrell failed to identify the variety of spokespersons of the various feminist groups. He also ignored those who deal with the problems of men that he cited (Hagan, 1992; Miles, 1991). Additionally, although this chapter does not presume to be a complete analysis of Farrell's work, he committed some glaring errors. In the introduction, he suggested that men do not express feelings because of an embedded fear of appearing weak to women. Research, however, consistently shows that men are much more willing to share feelings with women than with other men (Stewart, Stewart, Friedley, & Cooper, 1990). Hence, this problem does not seem to be an issue involving women, but a man's problem with other men. Although he discussed the predominance of men as victims of violent crime, he did not address the evidence that violent crimes against women continue to rise faster in the United States than any other country and that the "rate of violent crimes against women aged twenty to twenty-four has escalated by fifty percent in the last decade, while violent crimes against men in the same age range have decreased by twelve percent" ("So women are better off," 1992, p. 10). These data were available to Farrell who, apparently, chose to ignore them.

These three are significant and important books. They bring to light a great deal of information that may have been minimized by attention recently drawn to the condition of women in our society. Nevertheless, in their zeal to make men the victims, these writers create an unbalanced and biased portrait of the condition of men in the United States. Although their desire to achieve balance in attention to gender issues is laudable, they overlook the fact that personal or social equity between women and men in our society does not yet exist. Because this inequity is not even acknowledged, much less explored, the authors pass opportunities to develop communication strategies that would move gender relationships toward fuller mutual regard.

Although there are men's perspectives that are supportive of feminist positions (Kimmel & Mosmiller, 1992; Stoltenberg, 1989), the three reviewed books appear to be the most visible and dominant statements of a masculist point of view. What emerges from these three books are two specific major arguments from a masculist perspective. First, men need to delve into the unconscious corners of their own psyches in order to ferret out those insidious tumors that have caused them to shape their world in materialistic, combative, women-hating terms. Certainly, this is a viable and understandable concern and it is an area that clearly should be dealt with by men. A related second argument appears more dangerous and frightening: the claim, so clearly developed by Farrell, that the condition of men as powerless has been largely caused by women and, therefore, men must argue that their needs and wants are as important as women's. Putting the three writers' points together leads to the conclusion that women (in creating WOMAN) created the world that denies men their self knowledge, free choices, and the power of self control. Moreover, the claim is, this new men's point of view must be made as visible as women's before any real attempt at dialogue between men and women can occur.

This seems to create an incredible paradox: The assumption is that men, by discovering their wholeness, which is totally distinct from women, will then be able to relate to women more equally and fully. Yet, it is exactly those perceptions that have helped shape how men view women as significantly different and thus feed the inability to integrate masculine and feminine qualities. More recently, John Gray of "Mars and Venus" fame has also focused on differences between women and men, continuing to build the barriers and discouraging focus on integration of the feminine and masculine dimensions of human beings.

Would not men be more likely to develop a sense of understanding and equality if they spent more time doing more things with women, particularly in those arenas where there is a clear expectation of separation? From a prescriptive paradigm, an effective relationship would include the appreciation and acceptance of the similarities as well as the differences between masculine and feminine perspectives.

The examined books seem only marginally focused on understanding and developing ways for men to improve relational communication with women. In fact, the messages appear to encourage mistrust and defensive communication styles toward women, particularly in arenas where, by appearing weak (or "feminine"?) men may lose what little control they are being led to believe they have.

A contrasting voice, Faderman (1982) closed with this fantasy: "In an ideal world . . . men would not claim supremacy either in social or personal relationships, and women would not feel that they must give up a part of themselves in order to relate to men" (p. 415). Throughout, Faderman's point is deceptively simple; women and men should move to a perspective in which neither is superior, but both are equal, and the choices they make in personal and professional relationships are based exclusively on the individual needs of their own personalities. She appeared to state the perspective that most feminists (both women and men) would like to see develop: a sense of the equal[1]

---

[1]There is a continuing dialogue over the use of *equal* and *equitable* when referring to female-male relationships. One perspective is that it is not equality that is needed as much as equity—the move toward recognizing that women should have as much power in making and enforcing social rules as men have. A draft document (September, 1995) from the UN Women's Conference in Beijing stating that women have the right to refuse sex is an example of a statement of equity.

worth, value, and potential of all humans, regardless of gender. But such voices are not being heard. As mentioned in the beginning of this chapter, the movement toward gender equality in this country is currently slowed or halted, if not reversed. Too widely heard are the messages supporting that move, mostly from White men, reflecting the assumptions argued in the books I have just reviewed.

If men want to increase their awareness of the value of equitable relationships with women, they need to listen to and understand the women's' voices that tell us that sexual harassment occurs primarily in unequal power contexts; rape, including date rape, occurs because one person is stronger than the other and exercises that strength, which includes anger, hostility, and violence. Men need to understand that, compared to women of similar race and class, they have more power in most social, political, and professional contexts. They need at the least to recognize how those power relationships affect the interaction that occurs between women and men in those environments.

For men to "get it," at least intellectually, means that they understand cognitively what feminists, or, in fact, most women, are concerned with. To do that, they must hear women's voices. They can learn by reading feminist literature, by dialoguing with female friends and colleagues. They can read other men's work. A much less popular book than those reviewed here, more valuable in changing how men see women, is *Refusing to be a Man* (Stoltenberg, 1989). Stoltenberg confronted the basic elements that Goldberg (1987), Keen (1991), and Farrell (1993) appeared to want to perpetuate. He claimed that, for men, their biggest struggle is integrating information with attitudes and behaviors. He suggested that men should seek out continued interaction with women in ways that continue to move men and women toward equality of perceptions. None of the books reviewed here appear to do this. They offer a perspective of Man distinct, separate, and apart from Woman. It is maybe necessary for men to examine their own inner drives and male energies. Our culture and economic system is one, as Kimbrell (1995) discussed, that makes creating whole, healthy selves and psyches difficult for all its members, whether female or male. But to spend energy debating who is hurt worst, or how women have caused men' s problems, is to recreate old arguments long since left behind by most feminist writers.

For men to understand how they can improve their lives, they can at least attend to the way they relate to women, which requires hearing women's voices. What emerges from these three reviewed books, rather than an attitude of openness to women's voices, is a hostile and confrontive masculist voice that says: "let's make sure that men get all of their demands on the table and certainly do not admit that they, men, ever had any real power!"

In his book, *The Masculine Mystique,* Kimbrell (1995) created a "Manifesto for Men," in which he listed 19 goals that men should actively pursue to improve the masculine condition. Although including many laudable goals, not one indicates a way in which men can actively work toward more understanding of the feminine condition. In a subtle way, Kimbrell's message reflects the perspectives argued by Goldberg (1987), Keen (1991), and Farrell (1993). This continued resistance to hearing women's voices and attempting to diminish them rather than integrate them into our consciousness has already created a movement against women that Greenstein (1993) predicted will become much worse; "the human male is far more dangerous than I could ever have imagined, mainly because he does not understand just how dangerous he is" (p. 2). Although Greenstein's is a dire prediction, some evidence does support her scenario: the increasing physical violence against women, the increasing hostility against women's social and political concerns, and the failure of women to make significant gains in legislative and top managerial positions. Women's voices remain muted (Kramarae, 1981) and the major voices heard today are men who seem determined to maintain the illusion that they are really worse off than women.

It is appropriate to end by pointing out that there are men who hear and support women's issues. Authors such as Brod (1987), Kimmel and Messner (1992), Morris (1997), and Stoltenberg (1989) as well as organizations like the National Organization for Men Against Sexism have all expressed a recognition of the importance of hearing and actively supporting feminist perspectives. But their voices remain hardly a whisper as the shouts of the angry White males have become the dominant voice of the current backlash against women.

REFERENCES

Bly, R. (1990). *Iron John.* New York: Addison Wesley.

Brod, H. (Ed.). (1987). *The making of masculinities.* Boston: Allen & Unwin.

Brod, H. (1992). The mythopoetic men's movement: A political critique. In C. Harding (Ed.), *Wingspan: Inside the men's movement* (pp. 232-236). New York: St. Martin's Press.

Chappell, K. (1995, August). What they don't tell you about affirmative action. *Ebony,* 46-50, 135.

Cose, E. (1995). *A man's world: How real is male privilege—and how high is its price?* New York: HarperCollins.

Faderman, L. (1982). *Surpassing the love of men.* New York: William Morrow.

Faludi, S. (1991). *Backlash: The undeclared ware against American women.* New York: Crown.

Farrell, W. (1993). *The myth of male power.* New York: Simon & Schuster.

Goldberg, H. (1987). *The hazards of being male.* New York: Signet Books.

Goodman, E. (1991, October 12). Men are capable of "getting it." *Boston Globe,* C33.

Goodman, E. (1995, August 25). Secure to those who come after you . . . a larger freedom. *Los Angeles Times,* B9.

Greenstein, B. (1993). *The fragile male: The decline of a redundant species.* New York: Birch Lane Press.

Hagan, K. (Ed.). (1992). *Women respond to the men's movement.* San Francisco: Harper.

Keen, S. (1991). *Fire in the belly.* New York: Bantam Books.

Kimbrell, A. (1995). *The masculine mystique: The politics of masculinity.* New York: Ballantine.

Kimmel, M. S., & Messner, M. A. (1992). *Men's lives* (2nd ed.). New York: MacMillan.

Kimmel, M. S., & Mosmiller, T. E. (Eds.). (1992). *Against the tide: Pro-feminist men in the United States, 1776-1990.* New York: Simon & Schuster.

Kramarae, C. (1981). *Women and men speaking.* Rowley, MA: Newbury House.

Miles, R. (1991). *Love, sex, death and the making of the male.* New York: Summit Books.

Morris, L. A. (1997). *The male heterosexual.* Thousand Oaks, CA: Sage.

Reardon, K. K. (1995). *They don't get it, do they?* Boston: Little, Brown.

Renzetti, C. M., & Curran, D. J. (1993). *Women, men and society: The sociology of gender* (2nd ed.). Boston: Allyn & Bacon.

So women are better off today? (1992, July/August). *Peace and Freedom,* 26-27.

Stewart, L. P., Stewart, A. D., Friedley, S. A., & Cooper, P. J. (1990). *Communication between the sexes* (2nd ed.). Scottsdale, AZ: Gorsuch Scarisbrick.

Stoltenberg, J. (1989). *Refusing to be a man.* Portland, OR: Meridian.

Tavris, C. (1992). *The mismeasure of woman.* New York: Simon & Schuster.

Thomas, D. (1993). *Not guilty: The case in defense of men.* New York: William Morrow.

Wood, J. T. (1994). *Gendered lives.* Belmont, CA: Wadworth.

Yost, B. (1995, August 16). Backlash against women, minorities, is evident. *Fresno Bee,* B7.

17

MAGICAL VOICES

LEILANI COOK

Magical means "of or pertaining to magic," but what exactly is magic? *Magic* is a spiritual orientation that seeks to affect aspects of the material world by drawing on divine power. This rather ecumenical definition eschews the culturally biased debate about the differences between magic, science, superstition, and religion, and allows us to acknowledge that in various ways at various times, people seek to affect aspects of the material world by drawing on supernatural power. I present here two magical voices—a practicing Wiccan and a Catholic faith healer.

BOUND AND FOUND

The practicing Wiccan lives in a bright purple house by a large, spring-fed lake in northern Florida. The grounds are overgrown, except for a medium-sized, well-tended herb garden. Enjoying free run of the grounds are three large friendly dogs, and of course, the requisite inquisitive cat.

She is an imposing, articulate woman in her middle years, who earns her living by giving psychic readings, primarily through the use of Tarot cards. Although she is acutely aware of the historical dangers associated with being a witch, she does not keep her religious persuasion a secret. On her car are several humorous bumper stickers: "Honk If You Love Isis," "My Other Car is a Broom," "Magic Happens," and so on. Because of her openness, she has experienced a measure of harassment from members of the small, predominantly fundamentalist Christian community in which she lives who are unsympathetic to her spiritual orientation.

She came to Wicca as a convert. Her background is Reformed Jewish, and in fact, her brother has embraced Orthodox Hasidism, creating a polarity among the siblings that leads to "interesting times at Thanksgiving," as she puts it. She "worked alone" for a few years, but is now a member of a coven, which she much prefers.

In covens, she told me, the cooperative effort has a synergistic effect on the power raised to work magic, making the whole, so to speak, a product greater than its parts. Covens also provide comfort and psychological support to members in times of persecution, which appear to be, to varying degrees, all the time.

THE WICCAN SPEAKS

The following is transcribed from a lengthy interview on September 10, 1992.

> You want to talk about language, I mean there's so many words that were used to describe women, females, goddesses, that are considered weird words. Like "sinister" only meant left. Of course, if you use the word "sinister" now, people go, "Hmmmm . . ." And "gauche," means awkward, unsightly. "Oh my goodness! It's a real faux pas!" and again, left is all it means. Trivia—and who is more trivialized than women—was a goddess of information.
>
> Chaos is another goddess. She is so much the mother goddess with the aspect of Kali with the hands everywhere you know, cutting the threads and nothing makes sense, if you look at the beginning and the end and in a linear way, but chaos is very creative. Its got such a bad name because it seems like men don't have control. And that can make people hostile.
>
> That's why some of the charms that I have used most frequently of necessity have been around psychic attack. You know, someone that really decides to make a case against you somehow . . . or is out to get you. And its amazing how prevalent it is. Now sometimes you can

have your garden variety attacks, like an ex-husband, or wife, or lover, or something that just doesn't like where you're coming from and thinks bad thoughts about you all the time and wishes bad things. There's that, that's real garden variety and that happens to a lot of people. Or there's really foul-minded people who just sit around and want to dump on anybody, and you walk into a hospital or a courtroom or something like that and you're like aggggg! You know, deluged by negative vibrations, so I tell people, take a piece of black tourmaline which absorbs negativity, and that's one of the better charms I know for just absorbing negative energy. But one of the charms that I like an awful lot, that's been incredibly useful is the idea of using mirrors.

For instance, when there was a gang rape down in the fraternity houses here we led a silent vigil into the belly of the monster so to speak, wearing black and whiteface, and I brought a mirror with me, a round mirror about as big as a saucer, and I'm good at visualizing, but I found that literally using a mirror to bounce the energy back was so incredibly effective, plus it also adds a shock value, and people would start to stare at me, and it would remind me . . . boom. . . . Send it back. And many of the women who had gone on that particular action with me were vomiting and just really ill and upset and just really stretched to the max from the negativity that was just pouring on us by the frat boys just howling and yelling obscenities at us when we went through there to make a point.

The . . . [newspaper] got some pictures, actually. They've got a picture of us walking and the men on this truck making obscene gestures and ugly, contorted faces and really, the men showing their butts. But I felt fine after it 'cause the mirror bounced it back. We went in and we were silent, except sometimes we chanted part of a song written by Naomi Littlebear from Oregon, a chant that you can't kill the spirit.

Now a simple binding is good to prevent attack. I had a client, a neighbor here from the Black community and she was just having a really hard time. The landlord wanted to take the apartment back for someone in their family so they were doing everything in their power to make my client look bad so that she'd wind up losing her home, which she could not afford to have happen. So I said, OK, what you want to do, if you don't have a picture of the landlord, just take the name and write it down on a piece of paper, take some black thread, and wrap it all around, till you can't see the name anymore. And as you're doing that, you're thinking, "So may it be," you know, "So mote it be. I am binding your activities. No longer can you harm me and mine." And you bind them, you're just tying them up in their own web. The badness is all caught up—it's contained. And then you take the bound picture or name and you put it in a jar, and you put it in your freezer. I put it in a jar so it doesn't contaminate my food. It's real simple. I don't want it leaking. And I put it in the freezer just to chill it out. Just freeze its activity. And its really simple and its really effective, I find.

We did a binding on the Gainesville murderer. And, you know, the above ground activity was that I called all the women that I could think of and got us to march in the street, because the whole world was watching our community, and we wanted to say to the world that this violence against women has been around forever and we are aware that it is unacceptable, and that it is disgusting!

The underground activity was I called all the witches that I knew and we did a binding hex on the murderer by Lake Alice. Now Z[1] and I had hexed a gold-toothed rapist maybe 16 years prior, and 13 days later he was caught. So I decided we'd go back to a very lucky spot for women at Lake Alice and bind him so he couldn't escape and run away. And the words that we made up were, "May he be bound and found. Trapped by his own arrogance." I believe that what we did *did* stop something. No more bodies turned up, you know what I mean? Considering we were averaging one or two a day for a while, I'd like to think that it wasn't half bad.

The rule is, "Do what you will and harm none." We did not demand his legs be broken, or his prick to fall off, or him to die on the spot. We did a binding ritual, which does not invoke death or damnation, it invokes stopping the person. And that's really different. May the person be bound and found. So we took red cord around a black candle, and put urine on the black candle. Urine, menstrual blood, anything like that is considered powerful and we wrapped the red cord around the candle and thinking, and passing that around the circle, at a fever pitch, you know, "May he be bound and found, bound and found, bound and found." And, you know, passing that around. At that point I took a ritual knife and then I plunged it down into the earth to begin the binding and we worked with that and then we burned the candle way down to the ground. And after that night there were no more bodies found—by this particular killer, anyway.

A lot of times when I ask for certain things that I really need and I really want, they just sort of come. I've been living a sort of unconventional existence my whole working life. I've never done really a nine to five job, and yet, I've been able to support myself by my wits. Sometimes its been really edgy, but I always managed. And now I manage better.

SLAIN IN THE SPIRIT

October 15, 1993, I participated in a healing mass and faith healing service at a Catholic Church in northern Florida. The church was so new

---

[1] "Z" is Z Budapest, Flash Silvermoon's initiator into Wicca.

that parts of its parking lot were still unpaved. It was primarily plain and practical, but with some architectural touches that pleased the eye. The church's shape is that of a very scaled-down basilica, with rounded porticoes at both ends. No altar rail separates the altar from the nave; rather a series of low steps connects one to the other. This church was located somewhat far from the urban core, near other strongly charismatic and evangelistic Protestant churches.

The healing mass was a formalized ritual performed with sincere fervor by two priests, one saying mass, the other assisting. At the end of the mass, the priest said, "go in peace," and then, in the same breath, he said, "I don't want you to go," in a humorous tone, which provoked much laughter in the congregation because everyone knew they had all come to this mass as a part of a larger event (i.e. faith healing). Before the faith healer was introduced, one of the priests told of his sister's miraculous healing from glaucoma after her faith healing visit last year, and the other priest led the congregation in a song of welcome.

The songs were obviously selected for their highly emotive and simple qualities. For example, the welcoming song was entitled, "Yes, Lord, Yes," and its message was that when God calls followers must be ready to say "yes." The song established a context of openness to what was to follow. Saying "yes" is a big part of faith healing.

The faith healer was a middle-aged matron of Irish descent. Her speech was that of a midwesterner and she mentioned that she was from Chicago. She spoke to a microphone in a congenial, down-to-earth way, at first telling several well-known anecdotes about Saint Teresa of Avila whose feast day it was. After 30 minutes, when she was certain that she had acquainted everyone with the spiritual value and strength of Saint Teresa, she invoked this Saint to be with the congregation on this night. She also said that we would request the presence of the Holy Spirit and call it down to us for the purpose of healing and spiritual rejuvenation.

The congregation joined hands and sang two simple but lengthy hymns that had a mesmerizing, soothing, calming effect. Then the faith healer got down to business and asked the entire congregation to vocally and insistently praise Jesus in order to call down the power of the Holy Spirit. Here she began a speech pattern that was in very sharp contrast to the slow and peaceful chanting of the previous hymns. In a staccato measure she began to recite, and asked that we recite similarly, "We praise you Lord Jesus, we worship you, Jesus, we thank you, Lord Jesus, we glorify you, Jesus. We love you, Lord Jesus." These short sentences were repeated one after the other without any pause. The effect was like the rapid and continuous firing of pistons in an engine. People were not saying the same thing at the same time but they were chanting phrases of identical syntactic structure and semantic intent in an identical rhythm.

This chanting continued for approximately 15 minutes, and during that time the volume rose as the momentum increased. I felt very much like I was in a car listening to the revving of a powerful engine. During this entire time, without pausing for breath, the faith healer sustained her rapid-fire, rhythmically perfect chanting. Then, when she sensed that the appropriate level of heightened spiritual receptivity had been reached, and when she also sensed that the calling down of the Holy Spirit had been successful, she suddenly ceased speaking and announced, almost matter of factly, that she would begin the laying on of hands. She reminded congregation members that they must stay receptive and open to the power of the Holy Spirit. She exhorted people not to resist it, or shut parts of themselves off from it, but to let themselves go and trust God—and the "catchers" who were waiting behind each person.

At this signal, the congregation began to line up much as they had done to receive holy communion. The faith healer went from one individual to the next, always making some form of physical contact with each person before the actual laying on of hands and maintaining a running dialogue with each individual who came to the altar. She responded verbally to the statements and individual needs of each person. She embraced some people, whereas others she merely touched on the chest or shoulder. Then at the appropriate moment, she placed the palm of her hand on the forehead of the person who then fell backward, into the waiting arms of "catchers." This phenomenon is called being "slain in the spirit." The total physical relaxation after the laying on of hands of referred to as "resting in the spirit."[2]

THE FAITH HEALER SPEAKS

The following is transcribed from a lengthy interview on October 15, 1992.

> We were having a novena at our church and we invited a Redemptorist priest and when he came he prayed over me, along with everyone, and then I rested in the Holy Spirit and a nun came and prophesied and told me I had received the gift. It was in the person of our Lady.[3] She said, 'My dear little daughter, I bless you in a special way. I'm going to

---

[2]"Resting in the Holy Spirit" is the same as being "slain in the spirit."
[3]The Virgin Mary.

take care of your family and I have a new mission for you now with your gift of healing. And it was awesome . . . and I know that it was strangely true.

Sometimes if I go to a hospital and pray over one person I could walk out totally emptied. It's like that one person received everything. I guess it's like the Lord said: "I felt the power flowing through me. . . . I felt the power leave me." Sometimes I feel that during the service and I'll just have to stop and sometimes the Lord has to get my attention and sometimes I won't stop so then he really gets my attention, like Ugggh! I can't move! because this is the power of the Holy Spirit. It's tangible. It is a power. It's a substance. It's what the Lord wants to give to each person, and it's so individual. It's not a formula. And He lets me experience His love for each person, you know. And then I feel and I see . . . it's like I could see with a little bit of His eyes, with His heart. Like this kid came up to me at the end, you know, a big strong guy, and he says, I forget, but something like "What do you see in me?" And I said, "Goodness. Just goodness." And he says "What do you see in me?" and I says 'Jesus. That's what I see in you.' And essentially, that's it. The Lord enables me to see Himself in everybody. In a little baby it's the Lord. In the whole room it's the Lord, it's love. And you know, that's all that God desires for us. And it's all good will. He sees the good in us, and all the little acts of sacrifice and struggle in our lives. Like it says, "He was moved with pity for the crowd." He's compassionate. He wants to touch and free. It's all love. It's in no way like a condemnation. In fact it's like the worse the sinner, if we can make any judgements, the more the love. I'm just a channel for His infinite love. The mercy and love.

It stops and it starts, but it's always present, say like if someone called me on the phone and said will you pray, its right there. Its a gift, you know, its always available. Like someone called me from London when I first received the gift . . . years ago . . . and they wanted me to pray for this 19-year-old kid and she had gone to college and she was stricken with MS and she was totally paralyzed, the whole thing. And her family was so devastated and they asked me to pray for her. And I was going to mass and I said I'll pray for her, particularly at communion.' And I prayed for her, and then when I went to Ireland the next year they followed me all over giving the testimony, how right after, like within 24 hours she was up on her feet. 'Cause its the Lord who's the healer. I'm not the healer. He's the healer and that's why I don't really have to know anything.

I remember on one occasion I went to pray for this kid who was in a coma. And his dad was standing by the door. And I just prayed with the Dad and he just slithered down to the floor. There was no preparation, the dad didn't even know what it was. 'Cause the Lord is the healer. He knows it all, you know? You ask and you shall receive. Sometimes people will ask for someone else. And that's almost sure healing for them. When they think of someone else and they leave their own problems. When they say, "I'm sick but I want to pray for someone else" and then . . . they get healed.

But then some people don't even believe. Reporters usually ask me, "What would you say to the cynics?" And I say well, they become the biggest believers and promoters! Because they're credible! People will believe them because they had to be convinced. But then after a while they become incredible and we have to find new cynics. But the cynical and the hardened of hearts, the bitter, resentful, they'll come up, you know, someone got them there. And they're angry and . . . it's like they're saying, "Prove it to me!" And then, they go down. Arms folded, they're down![4] That's their woundedness, their scars, you see.

That prevents them from even hoping they could be changed, be healed or forgiven. Like the Lord wants to really give this one person something, like his love and his healing presence in a really dynamic way. And I'm like the mediator between them and Him and because of this love, He wants them to get it. Sometimes they'll say, "Well she pushed me down." Well, it could be. Maybe they're going to die in 2 days. Maybe this was their moment of grace and reconciliation and peace. He's offering them this gift!

The Holy Spirit does all the work. You know we had this real real big healing service in Chicago. There was about 1,000 people. And this guy, he was in a real severe depression and his friend had brought him. He said, "I gotta leave, I gotta go to work." And his friend said, "Oh, c'mon. Just let her pray over you." He hadn't ever seen it before. There was no preparation. And I laid hands on him and he went down. 'Cause the Holy Spirit will act and breathe where he will. Just like even resting in the Holy Spirit. It's a manifestation of the Holy Spirit, but you don't have to go down in order to be healed, you know. And sometimes when people don't even feel anything or experience anything they're healed anyway.

How do you block out the Holy Spirit? Sometimes people feel like it's so powerful. Like my organ player, she goes down like a cannon, it's just like a cannon when she goes down. It's this tremendous force. Like a cannon just shot you. She really goes down! And I can actually hear the poor guys behind her going "Uggh!" as she hits them. There's just this tremendous force. The Holy Spirit is life, you know, its his energy, his vitality. And that's what you're receiving.

---

[4]This reference is to the phenomenon of physical limpness common among recipients of the laying on of hands. Strong men volunteer as "catchers" during these ceremonies, standing behind the "slain in the spirit" and catching them when they go limp. Then they are gently laid on the floor of the church where they rest until they regain their physical composure.

COMMENTARY

These two women see their magical performances, and I think most people would also see them, in opposition, and they view each other with profound suspicion. To the Wiccan, who does not believe in Satan, Catholics represent the betrayal of the ancient pre-patriarchal goddess; a betrayal that led to the carnage of the crusades, the psychotic sadism of the Inquisition, and the current ecological rape of the planet. To the Catholic faith healer, witches are evil heretics who have been told about the true God but have chosen to worship his nemesis, Satan, instead.

The two magical performances have obvious differences. The faith healer is Christian, the dominant faith in the West. She performs before hundreds of people in the Catholic Church, a global organization of great power and prestige. She connects with her audience through the laying on of hands with a goal to start and spread something positive: the transmission of the Holy Spirit to the material world. Her audience approves; from the priest who introduces her to the congregation that approaches the altar, the participants in her public performance show support. Her public voice is loud and clear: She sings, tells anecdotes, affirms her faith, speaks to each seeker, and addresses her higher power, the Holy Spirit, and so on.

The witch, on the other hand, subscribes to a non-standard faith, one largely unacknowledged in this culture. She does not have the support of any large organization; in fact, her whole magical tradition eschews organization beyond the immediate level of a local coven. Rather than seeking connection, the wiccan seeks separation from her audience. She rebuffs it with her mirror, "bouncing the energy back," and her followers don whiteface and mime clothes, which set them apart. Her goal is to stop something negative: violence against women in a community nationally notorious for this phenomenon. Her audience often does not approve, so her magical performances are most often kept private—"underground." On the rare occasions when her performance is public, participants are hardly supportive. They include disapproving hecklers and overtly hostile reactions. Undoubtedly the biggest contrast, these interviews illustrate, is in their voice. In contrast to the faith healer's loud, clear public voice, the Wiccan performs a "silent vigil."

Although their voices seem to be at odds, these two middle-aged women have much more in common than either might readily admit. Both are professional channellers, in the sense that they see their life's task as channelling divine power to the material world, and both take donations for their services to subsidize their work. The Catholic faith healer channels divine energy from the Holy Spirit while the Wiccan channels equally divine energy, the "energy of the universe."

Both acknowledge as source of their special powers a female deity figure. The Wiccan's deity is the ancient Goddess; the Catholic's is Mary, the Goddess' surviving Christian counterpart.

The Wiccan tradition is oral while the Catholic tradition is predominantly written, but both draw on an ancient core of verbal lore, especially in channelling activities such as those reported here. The Wiccan cosmogony has a trinity of the three faces of the Goddess: Maiden, Matron, and Crone. The Catholic faith is also predicated on the concept of a trinity: Father, Son, and Holy Ghost. Wicca is polytheistic, but does have a concept of one ultimate creatrix of the universe. Catholicism is monotheistic, yet its hierarchy of saints and angels, who are seen as closer to divine than mortal, form a diverse pantheon.

The greatest similarity these women share, however, is the tendency of the larger society not to hear their magical voices. The Wiccan is clearly marginalized, but a closer look reveals that the faith healer is as well. Like many charismatic movements, the Catholic faith healer does not enjoy the unequivocal sanction of her church. Its support is understated: The mass was not offered during the prime Sunday morning hours, and information about the mass was disseminated entirely by word of mouth, reminding us of the Wiccan's reference to "above ground" and "underground" activities. Because their messages spring from a magical rather than an empirical tradition, both must confront, to varying degrees, "the cynical, the hardened of heart, the bitter, the resentful. . . ." Yet both women speak to profound needs and bring us their own truths. We would all do well to surmount our facile dismissal and hear the wisdom in their magical voices.

18

THE PATRIARCHAL CODE
WORKS AGAINST THE COMMON GOOD
OF ALL INDIVIDUALS

LOUISE GOUËFFIC

This chapter stands on the following premises:

I am a feme[1]   not a fe+male
  I am a fem   not a wo+man
    I am a sapien   not a hu+man
I can name my self, therefore, I am a namer, and therefore, I must be a critical thinker in the making of names, as well as in any other field of thought. It is my right as a namer to name myself; no one else can pretend to do so for me. To name me is to take my right of being a thinker away from me.

---

[1]The terms *feme* and *fem* are historical words and were borrowed into Middle English from French.

I came to this wisdom after I saw that I could not name the apple an *apfig*, because it would imply "figness" (i.e., an ap+fig), when one fruit was already named *fig*. Distinguishing class and member in the class has as much to do with the word created to communicate distinction as it has with the distinction that exists in reality. The word reflects reality. There is no figness in the object called an "apfig." Consistence is the heart of logic in naming reality. But this is not the case in the concept *mankind*.

This chapter is an analytical examination of patterns in words and sets of words in daily usage today—words that are based in the male being in his roles as man, father, husband, brother, and son, his semen and seminal potency—words used as the name of that which is the active principle of life and living. Although I use a few cross-cultural and intercultural examples, it is not an historical account of the phenomenon I discuss but rather a semantic and semiotic analysis involving the interlocking of meaning and symbol. The paradigm feature in this field of words is that the father is stressed as being the sole agency of thought and action because the principle of action is seen as being in the semen. For this reason, I call this field of words the *Patriarchal Code*.

The Patriarchal Code[2] consists of about 10,000 words in our current language that support man in his role as father-husband-man-son, as the basis of act, thought and reasoning, exposing the deep level structure of male bias or "sexism" found in language.

In this chapter I discuss the logical errors in the core of the Patriarchal Code discovered by the analysis of its core words, man, woman, female, and humanity, and so on, so as to get at the beams supporting and expanding the core. Although the core is not the issue in this chapter to provide the arguments exposing the basic paradigm, the patterns in the categories that support the core (i.e., the minor paradigms that reify the major paradigm).

Following are the arguments that expose the patterns.

First, the word *man* names the male **part** and the **whole** class: both the part and the whole are named man. If we accept this we also accept that "**man**" **is and is not male.** Ironically, at the same time, we accept that the distinction between part and whole is one of manness, when in the real world **to be man entails being male.** The magic wand of context is waved over this inconsistence to hide that man-the-male-part is man-the-whole-class. The nasty side of this is that because we did not know that we believed that *man is and is not male*, we trusted that man could name the part and the whole, which is why girls are easily

---

[2]See *Breaking the Patriarchal Code* (Gouëffic, 1996).

hooked into this code. The primacy of man as norm of the species is renewed everyday by the word *man*, part-and-whole.

The fig part does not constitute the whole of its class, and therefore, we cannot name the apple an *apfig*.[3] If we do we anonymize the apple, that is, we make it invisible as an apple. Anonymization of the other member in the class is precisely what happens in man part-and-whole in which to be man entails being male. To anonymize is to make invisible by denying the name.

Second, the word *man* is used to name the femininity-causing being wo+man, as if this being actually possessed manness, like the apfig possessed figness. The word *man* in wo+*man* helps to further "man is and is not male" while *to be man entails being male* remains in the real world. Manness has nothing to do with femininity cause. Adding "wo" to "man" does not change the necessity of maleness in being man anymore than adding ap to fig changes the necessity of figness for being fig. So what is the name of the femininity-causing being? . . . because wo+man is obviously not it. What little girls cannot put together because of their immaturity of thought processes is that wo+man is a man who is not a man. There is a good reason for this.

The word fe+male repeats the is-and-is-not-male, making it a pattern. The first thing a girl sees when she peeks into man's rationality bunker is that she is not male . . . and still included in man! To cover the fact that she is not male—and by now she's very confused—the word fe+male goes into her mind like ice cream goes into her belly. Because, as the apple is being transformed into a fig as an apfig, the girl is being transformed into a male who is not male by the word fe+male, which fits in neatly with the other illogical words, man, part-and-whole, generic man, mankind, and woman. In fe+male, the male part constitutes (the feme part) as not male. What is clever is that it is the truth that she is not male . . . and there is nothing so hard to find as a truth hidden in nebulous lies. If she is not male, what is she?

Third, the word hu+man covers all this inconsistence with an extra blessing. It does no harm to the man who is a man while transforming, once again, the man who is not a man into a man, and "includes" her in man as wo+man, while "to be man entails being male" stays in the real world. By now, I hope that you see that the only truth in

---

[3]How morphemes are put together, or left out, to name a concept becomes important to the task of giving a correct and convenient handle to a truth. For example, if we were to rename the apple an *apfi g*, by taking the sound "ap" in apple and adding "fig," and attempt to put this word into common usage, its acceptance would depend as much on putting *apple out* of usage. That is, it would depend as much on *making "apple" an absent word* as it would on putting the (false) word *apfig* into usage.

man-part-and-whole, generic man, mankind, wo+man, hu+man is **to be man entails being male**. This anonymizes fem and femeness, and what we are as a species, sapiens, old words that were currency long ago, but that have been put out of usage.

The matter, or concrete cause, which causes the effect of femininity, is **feme**, like the cause of masculinity is male. The feme animal who thinks (i.e., makes and uses words) is **fem**, like the male animal who thinks is man. When both respect the relations of cause and effect in themselves as self-reflective animals, that is, in—if boy (male) --> man, **then** girl (feme)-->fem-- we have wisdom, and this wisdom was long ago named **sapience**, whence the name sapiens.

This chapter cannot go into the etymological and historical events that show that the word *man* comes from a long process of subjugating the feme, and other males: Humanity is a concept that is linked to slavery and would make it linguistically legitimate. I no longer use the word: I call "humanity" the sweet euphemism for universal patriarchy. Anyone using these man-words words builds patriarchy anew everyday for the men who want the magic power in mind control over the species, slavery by another name. I say that I am in sapienity.

To return, then, to the topic of this chapter, I discuss some of the malicious paradigms found in the code which make the code convergenital[4] to language. Each example gives the patriarchal code word in bold followed by the role assigned to the feme or the word for feme in italics, with some comparative data where relevant.

1. **He is the namer, the signifier;** *she is the named,*
   man; *named fem 'wo+man'* (fem seen as object: she cannot name herself)
   Mr. Paul Jones; *names wife Mrs. Paul Jones*
   ander, Gr. man; *Andrea,ish,* Heb. man, *ishah,* etc.[5] (There are some 300 words that are based on this form.)
2. **He is the good, or perfect;** *she has value only through him*
   per[6] +fect -per, father + fect, made; *no equivalent* (absent word)
   per+ceive -father seeing; *no equivalent* (absent word), **per+mit,** etc. (Note that a giraffe does not do the act of perceiving. In the code there are several hundred words that claim the father as the basis of act, the subject of "verbe" [verpa L, verge, Fr

---

[4]Made by infixing *verge*, Fr., penis, L verpa, in *congenital, convergenital* means existing because of the penis.

[5]Hebrew is not an Indo-European language; nevertheless, wherever there is patriarchy there is a patriarchal code. The example is included here as analogy.

[6]Made by collapsing the p*t*r* formula to p*r as in par, meaning by (the father), in (the father), through (the father), etc., to convey that the father is sole subject of the verb and the head in social life.

penis]). Regarding the linguistic laws in the category of p*t*r* formula, which also make par and per as in parrain, godfather, and pere, as a different category morpheme, see footnote 6.

virtue -vir, L, man; *no equivalent*, etc. (There are some 400 words that are based on this form.)

3. **He is an individual;** *she is the collective or container*

    status, "us" denotes one (and male); data, "a" denotes feme and collective

    manus-L, hand, "-us" denotes male; *mana n/a*

    uterus - one organ; *mentula,* male sexual organs, more than one; etc.

    (cf. patrimony and matrimony). (There are some 2,000-3,000 words that show this genderization/personalization structure in "-us" versus "a.")

4. **He is mind (subject);** *she is body* (object), *working with object as "she"*

    God, the father, subject; (mother) *church,* (sister *ship*), object

    pilot, subject—male; *plane,* object—feminine,

    judge, subject—male; *justice,* object—feminine, etc. (Overlapping with 3, some 4,000 words are based on this structure.)

5. **He is the creator;** *she is the procreatress,* not co-creator

    God; *goddess, lesser god,* not a matter of male god and feme god

    anthropology, anthropos, man (male); *no equivalent*

    Paul; *Pauline, Paulette, Paula,* etc., the appended (to Paul) being, and thus lesser

    par+ent, par, father; no equivalent, silencing the mother's role, etc. (Some 700—800 words are based on this form.)

6. **He is divine;** *she is givine*

    The organs of the *mentula,* L, male genitals, are considered divine: it is a an Indo-European theological tenet that "the semen is the first principle of everything." The testes are theologically named "the living stones," and the erect penis is immortalized in the "divine phallus." None of the feme organs, not even the "birth canal" or vagina is considered divine; it is not given a theological name.

    It is important, then, to name the counterforce that goes to make people accept and then internalize the deeper message in the triad of living stones—divine semen—phallus. After prescribing "she" (to most objects), the belief is that "she" (the feme being) is passive and non-rational, and because she is passive she has the beautiful quality of **giving in** to what the mind-as-male says about her reality. To name this *"quality of* *giving in"* and to balance *divinity*, I made the word *givinity* out of "giving in." In this way, we can show the two forces at work: Divinizing the male genitals creates theology, the study of godman and givinizing the feme makes *sheology*, the study of femininity by observing objects such as ships, planes, mother nature, universities, (alma maters), mother church, mother earth, etc., objects designated as "she's," as the real *she* is designated as (sexual) object.

There are more paradigms in the Patriarchal Code, but this brief treatment offers a picture of the code as being a **code**, and a sense of how it works.

It is the repetition of the minor paradigms that causes through a cumulative process the psychological effect of belief in the major paradigm, that of father subject and mother object. I call this cumulative effect of the core and the paradigms *the common evil*. I do this to bring "the common good" into sharp contrast with it. Naming the evil made common through words as *common evil* gives contrast; everyone uses this biased language everyday, making us work as much for the common evil as for the common good. It splits the sexes into **Father Subject** (man-as-mind) and **Mother Object** (fem-as-body). This split, the *split-sex view* of self, splits mind and body without our knowledge. I call this part of the common evil, the *split-self view* of being, which fits hand in glove with the *split-level view* of nature and the world as supernatural (male) and subnatural (femeness as fe+maleness), with very little actually remaining natural. We are on a treadmill going nowhere fast.

I argue that if we look at the *whole* Patriarchal Code, more rational, more practical and more reality-based solutions suggest themselves. Looking at the so-called neutral term "chairperson" for a moment; it is supposed to be an improvement to "chairman." "Per" in person means father, and "son" is the base of sonality, sound or voice. There is no real improvement for anyone here; it felt like progress, not knowing that it was more of the same. Looking at the whole code brings such pitfalls into light. Indeed, the code, as a code of 10,000 words, suggested to me that we must rectify the naming of wo+man to **fem**, first, if we (fem) are to present ourselves as critical thinkers upon the world stage.

If we want to make real progress, and stabilize the progress, we are going to have to look at the whole Patriarchal Code to see how to rectify names, balance the situation in a rational and practical way and provide names for heretofore unknown phenomena such as givinity, sheology and the common evil. Right now, we can make an impressive jumpstart on this process just by calling ourselves fem, feme, and sapiens, for that is what we are. But we must also invent names and break into word-making in a radical way, with such terms as **fe+***male* "givinity" to explain how man canceled femness and expose how she was anonymized word by word.

In a chapter dealing with so few examples, the structure I am trying to convey may not be visible in its entirety. There are 10,000 words in the Patriarchal Code, the whole of which can be seen in *Breaking the Patriarchal Code* (Gouëffic, 1996). My insight after examining and seeing the whole Code is that *the reform of language has to take place before, or at least during, any other social, psychological, business, or other reform in order for the reform to be a practical and rationally-based one, one which creates real balance, and for the reform to achieve stability.* Suzette Haden Elgin also made a case for reform in language having to precede other reform at the Conference on Gender Research at Hollins College in spring 1992.

For instance, when you use *givinity* you are reforming language before social reform, because you must define the word when you use it. To do this you have to go into the major facets of cancelling femness: How objects are "she"; how she is a (sexual) object; how she is not allowed to name herself, justifying her quality of passivity; and how the girl internalizes this two-way passivity in "she"/she, and is then easily made to give in to all kinds of things (e.g., man calling her wo+man instead of fem . . . and, therefore, has this quality of givinity in her by man-made nature). If we do not have words with which to do good comparative work (i.e., naming givinity with divinity), we leave the code with thousands of clever tactics, but let the patrists always win . . . and fem and rational men, individually and collectively, always lose.

What is important to remember is: The cause of femininity is **feme**ness.[7] The feme animal who makes and uses words and speech to communicate is **fem**. She can be directly observed making and using words. As a fem **with** man, she is a sapien, a co-creator in the achievement of rationality and civilization. *First, there must be a consistent line of inference between the existence of the effect of femininity and the cause of this effect. Second, there must be a consistent line of inference between femininity-cause and the femininity-caused animal who learns to speak, think and ratiocinate.* If you do not follow cause and effect in yourself, you are presenting yourself as a nonthinker: you are not your own namer.[8]

---

[7]To see this cause and effect, it is necessary to go to observable entities. Maleness results in male concreteness, such that when maleness occurs then masculinity occurs. Maleness causes masculinity. Man has maleness. Therefore man causes masculinity. To be man entails being male.

[8]My book, *The Patriarchal Code*, exposes 10,000 terms showing the whole code and what is being done to the individual and collective mind. It took about 30 years to complete, and the book is as complete as it can be for now. I am happy to give it to my companion-sapiens only as a stepping stone for I realize that each chapter could be a book in itself. I leave it to fresh minds to bring fresh perspectives to the Code.

REFERENCES

Gouëffic, L. (1996). *Breaking the patriarchal code*. Manchester, CT: Knowledge, Ideas and Trends.

AUTHOR INDEX

SUBJECT INDEX

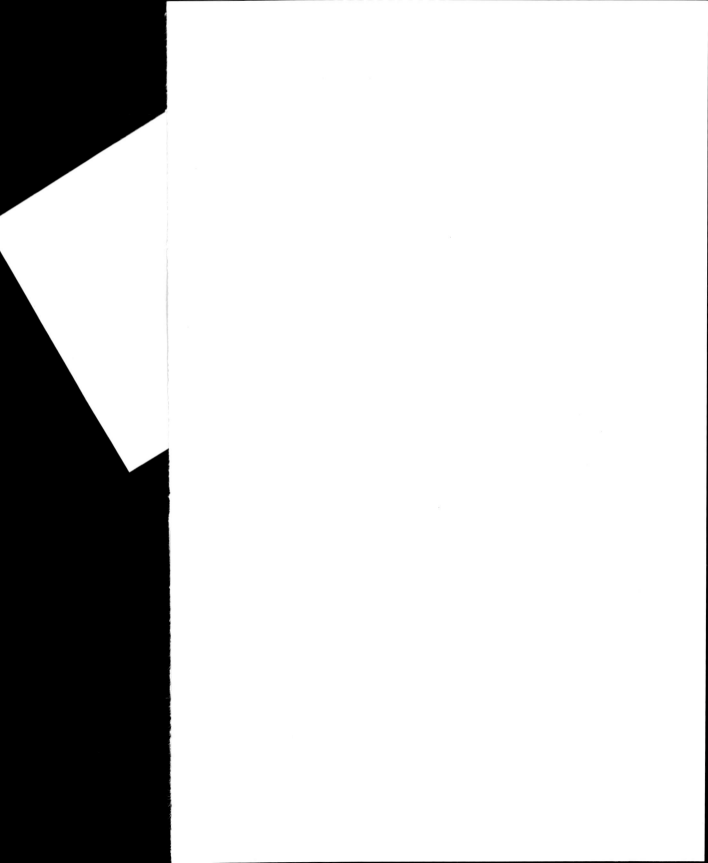

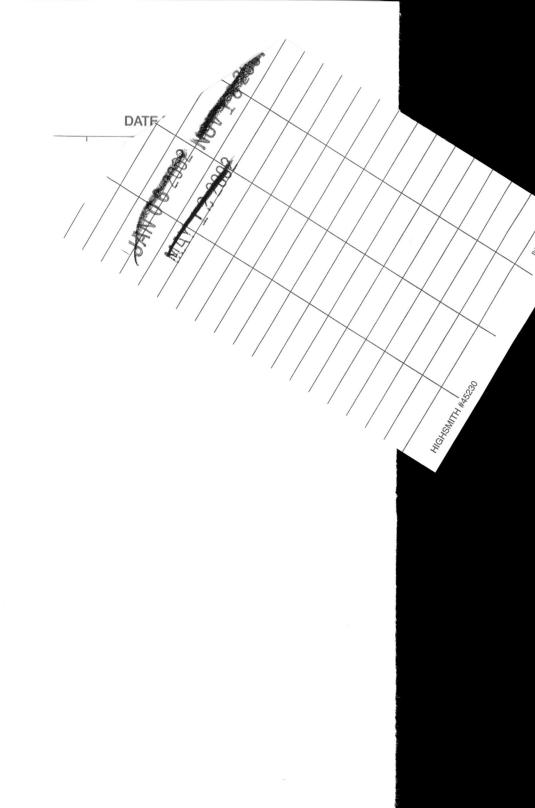

DATE

HIGHSMITH #45230

Printed
in USA